CHEST INJURIES

CHEST INJURIES

G. KEEN M.S., F.R.C.S.

Cardiothoracic Surgeon
United Bristol Hospitals and Frenchay Hospital
Clinical Lecturer in Thoracic Surgery
University of Bristol

Second Edition

WRIGHT
BRISTOL
1984

Published by
John Wright & Sons Ltd., 823–825 Bath Road, Bristol BS4 5NU
England

First edition, 1975
Second edition, 1984

British Library Cataloguing in Publication Data

Keen, G.
Chest injuries.—2nd ed.
1. Chest—Wounds and injuries
I. Title
617′.54 RD536

ISBN 0 7236 0815 6

TYPESET BY BATH TYPESETTING LIMITED

PRINTED IN GREAT BRITAIN BY
JOHN WRIGHT & SONS LTD., AT THE STONEBRIDGE PRESS, BRISTOL

Preface to the First Edition

This book is addressed to general surgeons, accident surgeons and anaesthetists who are those responsible for much of the primary and subsequent care of patients with chest injuries. It is fortunate that the majority of patients respond favourably to measures well within the competence of those who staff our accident units, for these injuries frequently occur in areas remote from hospitals staffed by thoracic surgeons.

The advice contained in these chapters is based on my own experience. I am aware that there are many pitfalls of diagnosis and treatment that are responsible for avoidable complications and deaths. Not all thoracic surgeons and anaesthetists will agree with all the views expressed here. Nevertheless, I hope that they will find this book helpful and I know that they will see that it will also be a practical guide for those who find themselves dealing with a case that is outside their experience.

The early chapters consider the general principles of diagnosis and management, many of the methods described being familiar. Although specific problems are conveniently described in separate chapters, it is recognized that several injuries may occur together in the same patient. Some injuries, particularly traumatic haemothorax and flail chest, are common, whereas others such as traumatic rupture of the bronchus may rarely be encountered. Nevertheless, full discussion of uncommon injuries and of iatrogenic injuries of the oesophagus is not considered out of place.

G. K.

Preface to the Second Edition

Since the publication of the first edition of this book 10 years ago, the prognosis of patients with serious chest injuries has considerably improved. This is due more to advances in the management of critically ill patients than to any particular improvements in techniques of the care of chest injuries. Over this period more hospitals have established active and effective intensive care units and a greater number of doctors and nurses are now very well trained in the management of these patients. Consequently the commonest causes of death following chest injuries, which are anoxia and haemorrhage, are less likely with the more effective management of the airway and the pleural cavities, and the realization of the importance of fluid and blood replacement in adequate amounts where appropriate.

The controversy concerning the relative merits of intermittent positive pressure ventilation versus surgical stabilization of fractured ribs in the treatment of flail chest remains unresolved, although the indications for the latter procedure in experienced hands are more clearly defined.

The increasing use of continuous epidural analgesia in the management of chest injuries has reduced the need either for internal fixation of fractured ribs or for prolonged intermittent positive pressure ventilation and the important place of the intensive care anaesthetist in the management of chest injuries is acknowledged.

Although the recent introduction of SI units is gradually gaining acceptance in hospitals in the United Kingdom, it is clear that at present the majority of hospitals and intensive care units have not adopted SI units when measuring blood gases. Consequently, the measurement of blood gases with reference to partial pressures is retained in this edition.

G. K.

Contents

Chapter 1

Introduction

In no field of surgery is it more essential to observe the time-honoured principle that diagnosis precedes treatment. When a seriously injured patient is admitted to hospital it is necessary to diagnose the full extent of the injuries and then to undertake such first aid treatment as is necessary to keep the patient alive. The selection of priorities for the definite treatment of these injuries may tax the wisdom of the most experienced general surgeon and his specialist colleagues, and the role of the accident surgeon is therefore not a happy one. His task is certainly lightened by instruction in diagnostic procedures, the basic principles of management, and simple resuscitative surgical techniques.

It is probably the case that most fatal mistakes in the early management of chest injuries result from errors in diagnosis, or from incomplete diagnosis. Unfortunately, the diagnosis and treatment of chest injuries is not well taught, if taught at all, in our medical schools; nor is practical instruction given in the minor surgical techniques involved in the first aid management of these cases. This is a pity, for these surgical techniques are relatively simple to apply when the correct diagnosis has been made. The aim is to maintain a clear airway, to relieve pulmonary compression by air and blood, and to sustain the mechanical respiratory efficiency of the thoracic cage. The surgical repair of injuries to the heart, aorta, bronchi, oesophagus and diaphragm is a procedure that may frequently be delayed until resuscitation has been achieved and the patient's condition has stabilized. It is at this point that consultation between the thoracic surgeon and his other surgical colleagues will determine whether thoracotomy should be performed before, synchronously with, or after their surgical procedures.

The majority of patients with chest injuries remain under the care of general surgeons, few being admitted to thoracic surgical centres, with consequent widely varying standards of management related entirely to the experience of those at hand. Although an increasing number of doctors and nurses have the opportunity to gain experience of thoracic surgery, there is little doubt that an aura of mystery seems to surround the injured chest wall and its contents. Experience of this unsatisfactory state of affairs suggests the need of a clear understanding of the management of these injuries. It seems inevitable that despite greater specialization and improvement in standards of patient care, few of these patients will be seen by a chest surgeon and it therefore falls to others to manage treatment: these are general surgeons, orthopaedic and accident surgeons, and anaesthetists. They have in common a primary interest in their own specialty or their own part in the treatment of the patient, the degree of priority given to the chest injury being related to the severity of associated injuries and the interest and experience of the doctor.

The increase in road traffic accidents has been accompanied by a parallel increase in severe injuries of all kinds, among which chest injuries are prominent and often fatal. The majority of patients with a chest injury have associated injuries. Head injuries, abdominal injuries or major fractures are usually obvious or at least seriously suspected, and the general surgeon or appropriate specialist will see the patient with little delay. Less happily, those with serious and perhaps fatal chest injuries may have little or no outward evidence of such damage with consequent delay in diagnosis, during which dangerous anoxia may develop or serious bleeding continue. Such injuries are frequently missed because chest radiography has been considered unnecessary. Standard physical examination of the chest, although essential, can be most deceptive and there is no substitute for a chest radiograph.

It is estimated that 30 per cent of those injured patients who die before reaching hospital do so because of chest injuries, and in a further 20 per cent chest injuries significantly influence the fatal outcome, suggesting that up to one-half of traumatic deaths are due directly or indirectly to chest injury. Others die shortly after admission to hospital, but of the remainder most should survive for in these the journey to hospital and the delay within the hospital constitute a robust test of survival. However, many of these patients do not survive and some of the reasons for this may become clear as various chest injuries are discussed. This is a gloomy picture, for the majority of chest injuries are not intrinsically fatal and with prompt and appropriate attention far fewer should die. Although ambulance teams receive increasingly effective training and may include a doctor, it is unrealistic to expect that loss of life at the roadside or during transport to hospital can be significantly reduced. More, however, could be done for those who arrive alive.

Closed trauma accounts for the great majority of chest injuries in this country, and road traffic accidents are the primary cause. The mortality of isolated closed chest injuries is about 10 per cent, increasing to 15 per cent when another system is involved. In the event of involvement of two other systems in addition to the chest injury, a mortality of 25 per cent is likely. Particularly lethal is the combination of chest and head injuries whereas associated limb injuries and fractures are better tolerated. The mortality rate rises rapidly with increasing age and most published series confirm this especially after the sixth decade. Coexisting cardiac and respiratory disease doubtless influence the outcome in the elderly.

Chapter 2

Assessment of patients with chest injuries

Patients with chest injuries are best observed in the intensive care unit where nurses familiar with techniques of resuscitation are available and a resident doctor is at hand. Such units will be equipped with adequate patient monitoring apparatus and the wherewithal for respiratory and circulatory resuscitation. This combination of the right people and the right equipment is concentrated at no other part of the hospital and the intensive care unit offers the most favourable environment for survival. Frequent examination of the patient is complemented by the use of a progress chart and it is useful to record the following measurements at frequent intervals.

ARTERIAL PRESSURE

In most cases recording of the blood pressure using a sphygmomanometer cuff will be adequate. However, in the seriously injured, who may have marked peripheral vasoconstriction, direct recording of the arterial pressure using a radial artery cannula may be of great assistance. This requires the use of transducers and electro-manometric equipment, together with personnel trained in their use. Certainly, in those units where such apparatus is in constant use great benefit is to be derived from these observations. Furthermore an arterial cannula gives ready access for arterial blood gas estimation.

CENTRAL VENOUS PRESSURE

When dealing with the seriously injured or those in a state of surgical shock monitoring of the central venous pressure should be accepted as a routine procedure. The catheter may be introduced by way of an arm vein or by percutaneous puncture of the internal jugular vein or subclavian vein, the catheter tip being placed in the superior vena cava. Radio-opaque catheters are useful for there is then no doubt that the appropriate vein has been entered. A simple water manometer is adequate and accurate, electro-manometry being a luxury. It is, however, important for staff to understand that since low pressures are involved a standard point be chosen on the chest wall as the zero measurement, for variations in the patient's position will otherwise produce apparently bizarre readings. It matters little whether the chosen point is the sternal angle or the anterior axillary line, so long as it is constant for that patient. Such a cannula will also serve as a reliable route for rapid blood transfusion and for the infusion of irritant liquids, such as concentrated sugar solutions, which might otherwise cause thrombosis of peripheral veins.

Intelligent assessment of the significance of arterial and central venous pressures will help in the estimation of blood loss or continued blood loss and furthermore may give information concerning the development of pericardial tamponade, cardiac failure or of over-transfusion.

URINARY CATHETERIZATION

It is wise to catheterize the bladder of all seriously injured patients for urinary output may reflect the degree of hydration and perfusion of the patient.

BLOOD GAS ANALYSIS

A serviceable well-maintained apparatus for blood gas analysis, together with an experienced operator, is an essential tool in the assessment of patients with chest injuries. Not only will frequent estimations of $P\text{ao}_2$ and $P\text{aco}_2$ indicate the adequacy, improvement in or deterioration of ventilation but measurement of the blood pH will indicate in many instances the state of tissue perfusion.

RESPIRATION

In addition to frequent measurements of rate, note should be made of the type of respiration and whether it is associated with straining, tracheal tug or indrawing of the chest wall, for these signs of ventilatory insufficiency must be recognized early. In those who have undergone tracheal intubation frequent assessments of tidal volume using a flow meter will be valuable.

Consideration of these observations will indicate a stable state or a trend towards improvement or deterioration. In selected units computerized control of these measurements is on trial with early encouraging results, trends being predicted by the computer in some cases well before staff are aware of such changes. There is no substitute, however, for constant clinical examination supplemented by frequent chest radiographs.

CAUSES OF EARLY DEATH

Anoxia and bleeding are the primary causes of early death and may be associated with one or more of several readily recognized conditions:

Airway obstruction
Tension pneumothorax
Haemothorax
Flail chest
Pericardial tamponade.

These may be recognized by clinical examination supported by radiography and it cannot be over-emphasized that chest radiography is an important part of early assessment. This should not mean that the patient is taken to the X-ray department by a porter with a request form, for radiographers and other technical staff in the X-ray department are in no position to decide on priorities. It is under such circumstances that from time to time sick patients become critically ill while waiting in the queue.

The portable machine and its operator should be immediately available by the bedside, for with pneumothorax, haemothorax, atelectasis or ruptured diaphragm minutes may be vital. Assessment of airway obstruction is not difficult, the force, duration and frequency of breathing and the presence of stridor being noted, and movements of the chest wall being observed. Inspection of the chest wall will show whether or not both sides move well and equally and a flail segment may be obvious. Tracheal tug and indrawing of the costal margin are features of airway obstruction and should be sought in all cases. Percussion and auscultation of the chest may show evidence of pneumothorax or haemothorax. Examination of the neck may show tracheal deviation due to tension pneumothorax and, although distended neck veins are commonly seen with straining or violent patients, their persistence after sedation might indicate cardiac tamponade.

Surgical emphysema will be obvious and, if of rapid onset and rapid progression, may give rise to suspicion of rupture of a major air passage.

The weak rapid pulse of blood loss contrasts with the full bounding pulse of CO_2 retention, and the paradoxical pulse of pericardial tamponade may be recognized and associated with a stab wound of the chest or upper abdomen. Relative weakness of femoral pulses or of the pulses in one arm may suggest aortic or subclavian artery damage.

Anoxia and Hypercapnia

Anoxia may be caused by haemorrhage, collapse of lung due to pneumothorax, haemothorax or an obstructed airway, pulmonary contusion or be due to inadequate ventilation. As with bleeding, the diagnosis of anoxia may be difficult and consequently be delayed until a late and perhaps terminal stage. These difficulties are encountered not only by junior staff but have caused embarrassment to experienced observers. Poor or artificial light may readily deceive, and even in good light the assessment of the degree of cyanosis varies from observer to observer. Pallor due to haemorrhage adds to these difficulties. A good bedside assessment of cyanosis is the direct comparison of the examiner's and patient's nail bed when viewed in good light, and with experience significant cyanosis is readily noted.

However, in addition to anoxia, carbon dioxide retention may coexist and this is less readily diagnosed by the bedside. Observation of the patient's breathing is important, the rate and depth giving some indication of efficiency, although in the unconscious these features may be misleading. Ineffective respiratory efforts associated with indrawing of the costal margin may indicate respiratory obstruction. The most accurate method of assessing the degree of anoxia is that of blood gas analysis and facilities for immediate and accurate measurement of arterial oxygen and carbon dioxide tensions and arterial blood pH should be available close to the accident unit. Not only do such measurements indicate the adequacy of ventilation and perfusion, but repeated estimations will help assess the value of treatment or indicate deterioration.

It is unfortunate that dangerous anoxia is not necessarily associated with either shortness of breath or obvious cyanosis. A tension of 60 mmHg Pao_2 is the equivalent of about 90 per cent saturation of haemoglobin with oxygen but is nevertheless entering a dangerously low level and further anoxia may lead to cardiac arrest. Consideration of the dissociation curve of oxyhaemoglobin demonstrates that below a level of Pao_2 of 60 mmHg oxygen saturation falls off extremely rapidly (*Fig.* 1).

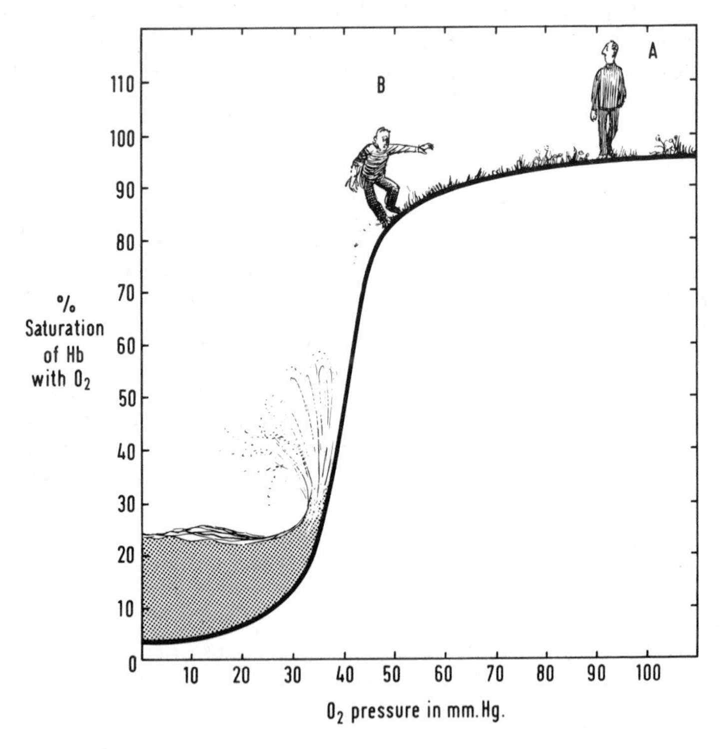

Fig. 1. An arterial oxygen tension of 60 mmHg should be viewed with extreme caution.

Blood Loss

Estimation of the extent of blood loss may be difficult, the more so in the absence of external wounds. Several litres of blood may be lost into the chest wall and pleural cavities, and intra-abdominal bleeding or the haematoma which surrounds major fractures can significantly increase this loss. In the young and previously healthy the peripheral circulation and cardiac reserve can mask a serious decline in blood volume until a near-terminal state has been reached, blood pressure and pulse rate remaining remarkably normal. Although pallor, sweating and other classic signs of bleeding may be present, the absence of these features is by no means rare, especially in the unconscious or those adequately sedated.

Consideration of the whole clinical picture, together with central venous and arterial blood pressure measurements, may give a fair indication of the patient's blood volume, and furthermore may indicate continued hidden blood loss.

FURTHER CARE

Once the patient's condition has stabilized and the airway and ventilation are adequate, blood loss may be replaced and pneumothorax or haemothorax be attended to. By this time other injuries have been assessed by appropriate specialists and the order of priority of their treatment discussed. It is as well to undertake as many procedures as possible under one anaesthetic, although this should not be overdone. Certainly, in the presence of a serious chest injury simple skin traction or back slab plasters will suffice for the majority of fractures, as a delay of several days before operative reduction and fixation is well tolerated. Intra-abdominal injuries necessarily require early laparotomy and the neurosurgeon may find himself forced into early craniotomy.

Although the immediate chest problem may be under control the possibility of other dangerous and as yet undisclosed chest injuries should now be considered. Giving rise to perhaps surprisingly few symptoms and signs at the time of admission, closed aortic rupture, ruptured diaphragm, ruptured oesophagus, severe lung contusions or closed intracardiac damage may be associated with a later sudden but serious deterioration, leaving little time for diagnosis and treatment.

Consequently, before discharge from the special care unit to the general wards, full further clinical evaluation and perusal of further good quality radiographs are necessary. Once he has returned to the general ward the patient is very much on his own, and having been pronounced fit by the doctors in the intensive care unit may place him at great risk for in the eyes of his new guardians deterioration or further setbacks may not be anticipated. It is important that continuity of medical care follow the patient from the time of admission to discharge. The practice of one group of doctors controlling the special care unit in isolation from others is prevalent but not recommended. There is little point in physicians and surgeons complaining about the standard of management of their patients in these units by others if they apparently have neither the time nor inclination to visit this ward. The management of patients in any intensive care unit is an exercise in communication and diplomacy, and many problems which arise can be traced to failures here.

Great credit is due to the brave attempts, although sometimes amateur, by special care doctors to manage these patients alone. It is under such circumstances, however, that patients may have less than the best at our hands.

Chapter 3

Management of pain

The pain of chest injuries may be severe enough to interfere with ventilation and coughing, perhaps prejudicing survival. Deep breathing and coughing are avoided and hypoventilation with sputum retention may pose a serious problem. Attempts to encourage the patient to cough may be unsuccessful until adequate analgesia is forthcoming. This derives from the understandable but incorrect view concerning the deleterious effect of analgesic drugs on the patient's ability to cough and breathe, with consequent denial of pain relief. There is little doubt that with appropriate drugs and techniques much of the pain of these injuries can be relieved.

ANALGESIC DRUGS

Although simple analgesics may help many forms of pain they are of limited value in controlling the severe pain of broken ribs. Morphine and its derivatives have acquired a bad name in chest surgery because of their known respiratory depressant effect. However, when used in small incremental doses intravenously, morphine is of great value. The patient becomes relaxed and co-operative with obvious improvement in ventilation and coughing. Alternatives in the form of synthetic analgesics may from time to time give adequate pain relief but their effect is often disappointing.

LOCAL ANALGESIA

The injection of local anaesthetic agents either locally into the site of rib fractures or regionally has gained wide acceptance and in skilled hands may deal effectively with chest pain. This not only helps pain-free coughing but enables sedative drugs to be reduced in dosage. A safe local anaesthetic agent is lignocaine hydrochloride and up to 25 ml of a 0·5 per cent solution may be safely used in adults. It is of interest that the pain relief consequent on injection of this drug may last for a far greater time than its known effect when used elsewhere, and this treatment may be repeated when necessary. A very useful long-acting local anaesthetic is Marcain (bupivacaine) which may give pain relief for as long as 12 or 15 hours. Although pain relief may be excellent, precise local injection into the site of rib fractures may be difficult to achieve for the region may be oedematous and contused.

REGIONAL ANALGESIA

Intercostal Nerve Block

This is an effective method of controlling the severe pain of broken ribs and when successful such a nerve block improves the patient's condition and confidence in a most acceptable way. The intercostal nerves are best blocked just lateral to the paravertebral muscles. A subcutaneous weal of local anaesthetic is first raised at each injection site. The anaesthetic is injected just beneath the rib and after aspiration to ensure that a vessel has not been entered and the pleura has not been penetrated. It is usual to block the nerves of the fractured ribs and to include one or two nerves above and below. Although it is theoretically unwise to block more than six intercostal nerves for fear of paralysing the chest wall, such fears are groundless for with unrelieved pain reflex spasm renders the chest immobile in that area (*Fig*. 2).

Continuous Epidural Analgesia

This has the advantage that once a fine catheter has been introduced into the epidural space by the anaesthetist repeated injections produce prolonged periods of analgesia. Although pain relief is excellent the associated sympathetic blockade may, in the elderly, produce an undesirable fall of blood pressure. Such hypotensive episodes should be taken seriously for in predisposed patients cardiac arrest or cerebral thrombosis may follow. If, therefore, following epidural block in an elderly patient, significant hypotension occurs the procedure should be reviewed and the blood pressure encouraged to return to normal by the use of plasma expanders.

INHALATION ANALGESIA

Despite the widespread and satisfactory use of self-administered nitrous oxide in obstetrics, its qualities have been insufficiently

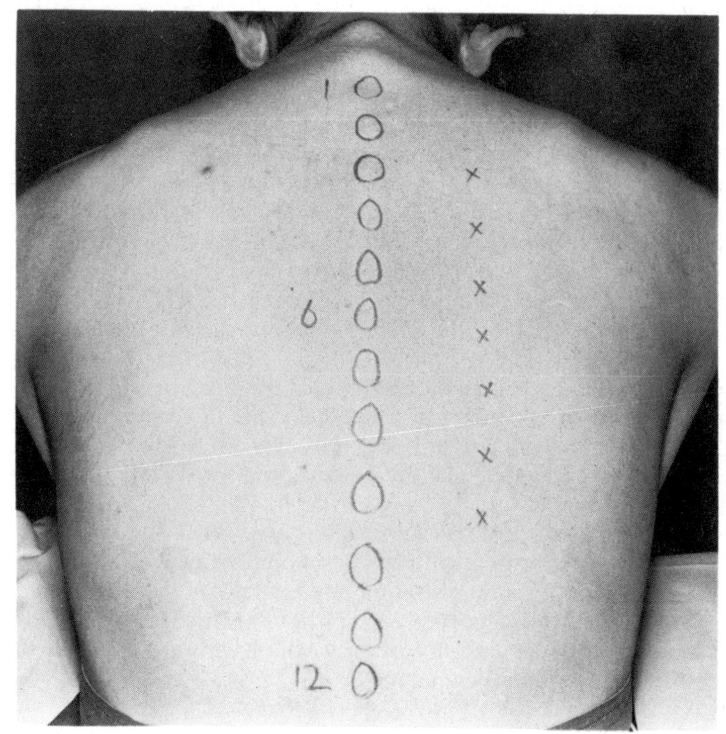

Fig. 2. Sites of election for intercostal nerve block with fracture of ribs 4–8 on the right side. Block of the intercostal nerves above and below the injury is recommended.

exploited in other branches of medicine. Doctors and nurses daily inflict avoidable pain on numerous patients, analgesia being denied because the procedure is deemed minor or the pain considered trifling. Denial of analgesia is often with the good reason of caution or the less good reason of inconvenience to staff.

Entonox, a mixture of 50 per cent nitrous oxide and 50 per cent oxygen, is a safe, effective general analgesic of rapid onset which is rapidly eliminated. Nitrous oxide is a powerful analgesic and sedative which if given with oxygen causes neither cardiovascular nor respiratory depression. Entonox is a stable gas even when compressed to 2000 lb psi. It is administered utilizing the demand or intermittent principle, the gas not flowing unless a negative pressure is applied to the inspiratory port. This requires an airtight fit between the mask and face, a conscious effort of the patient being required to ensure adequate gas flow. This safeguards the patient from a relative overdose and he is prevented from entering the uncooperative phase of general analgesia. The use of Entonox is approved by the Central Midwives Board for use by medically unsupervised nurses and midwives, and is also approved by the Department of Health for use by unsupervised ambulance crews. It is particularly suited to otherwise painful chest physiotherapy, for it has been shown that during its use not only is ventilation and coughing greatly improved but $Pa\text{O}_2$ levels rise considerably (Baskett and Bennett, 1971). When used in chest injuries the relatively pain-free and co-operative patient has less chance of developing the more common complications of pulmonary collapse and sputum retention.

Entonox has been used successfully in conjunction with artificial ventilation for many hours at a time, the safe upper limit being as long as 24 hours of continued administration. Such patients are sedated but co-operative and are able to cough well helping to clear their secretions.

In any particular unit no one method will prove suitable for all patients but a judicious combination of morphine, regional nerve blocks and Entonox administration proves useful in the management of chest injuries. It is important for a positive attitude to be developed on the part of nurses and doctors if we are to give our patients the safe pain relief which they require.

Chapter 4

Management of the airway and of ventilation

Airway obstruction is a common cause of death following injury, particularly in the unconscious. Such obstruction may be due simply to posterior displacement of the tongue which is readily relieved by elevating the jaw forwards and the introduction of an oropharyngeal airway. Ambulancemen and first-aiders are well trained in the recognition and treatment of this dangerous situation but nevertheless patients frequently die of asphyxia shortly after injury.

Following admission to hospital retention of secretions may become a serious problem. The capacity of the trachea and major bronchi is less than 50 ml in an adult and far less in children, and it is clear that small volumes of mucus, pus or blood can cause significant and perhaps dangerous airway obstruction. Furthermore, vomiting with aspiration of food, beer and gastric juice commonly accompanies chest injuries and this aggravates the problem. Recognition of such obstruction is frequently delayed, the more so in those whose coughing and level of consciousness are impaired. At bronchoscopy it is not uncommon to find the trachea and major bronchi awash with mucus, food debris and blood, and it is surprising that respiratory exchange is possible under these circumstances. Airway obstruction is far less of a problem in the conscious and co-operative, but in the semi-conscious, unconscious, disorientated and intoxicated sputum retention is common. Furthermore, chest pain or interference with the integrity of the chest wall in turn impairs effective coughing.

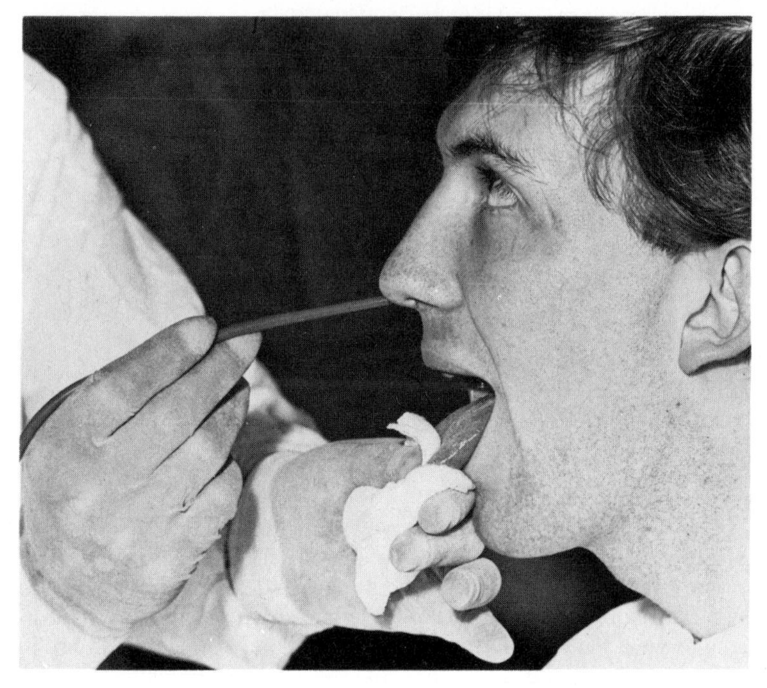

Fig. 3. The ideal position for effective nasotracheal suction.

PHYSIOTHERAPY

This is the most important primary method of managing the airway and of dealing with sputum retention. The availability of round-the-clock physiotherapists skilled in the care of chest injuries may mean the difference between good co-operative airway clearance or the necessity to resort to bronchoscopy or tracheostomy. For the physiotherapist to succeed the patient's confidence must be gained and here pain relief is of great importance. The days of robust therapists treating frightened patients who are in pain are largely behind us but this is in part a consequence of our better understanding of the use of pain relief. It is held by some that sedation is dangerous on account of depression of the respiratory centre but more damage results from sputum retention than from sedation administered in appropriate doses at regular intervals.

Physiotherapy sessions are best preceded by a period of postural tipping to allow the affected lobe or lung to drain into the central air passages. This is followed by the attention of the physiotherapist and it is then that pain relief is necessary.

Nasotracheal Aspiration (*Fig.* 3)

Despite seemingly adequate physiotherapy, sputum retention may occur, recognized by examination of the chest or producing radiological evidence of segmental or lobar collapse. In these patients the introduction of a fine suction catheter through the vocal cords will produce forceful coughing enabling peripheral secretions to be moved more centrally, whence they are readily aspirated.

The patient should sit up at 45°, the tongue firmly grasped with a gauze swab and drawn forwards. The neck should be flexed forwards on to the chest, but the head extended at the atlanto-occipital joint. In this position with the tongue held well forwards and with the patient taking deep breaths, a lubricated catheter introduced into the nostril will usually find its way through the vocal cords and into the trachea, this manœuvre being rewarded with productive coughing. Should coughing not follow, asking the patient to speak will confirm the whereabouts of the catheter; if between the cords the voice is characteristically altered. In such circumstances the instillation of 5 ml of saline through the tube may induce coughing. It is important that suction is not applied to the tube for long periods to avoid hypoxia. Rotation of the head from one side to the other may enable the bronchi to be separately entered.

BRONCHOSCOPY

This procedure is more commonly reserved for injured patients able to cough but whose secretions are too thick to respond to nasotracheal aspiration. General anaesthesia should be avoided for it is important that a physiotherapy session should follow bronchoscopy. Local anaesthesia is adequate and atropine is administered half an hour prior to bronchoscopy. With care the risk of bronchoscopy in these patients is negligible. Bronchoscopy is best undertaken with the patient sitting up in bed at an angle of 45°, the operator standing on a platform behind the bed. Although the majority of patients respond well to one or two bronchoscopies, it is important to avoid frequent repetition of this procedure for even in the most experienced hands some degree of trauma to the vocal cords is inevitable, and, furthermore, bronchoscopic aspiration is a harrowing experience for the conscious patient.

The flexible fibreoptic bronchoscope is of great value in this situation and in some centres has superseded the use of the rigid bronchoscope.

TRACHEAL INTUBATION

When it is clear that despite adequate physiotherapy, naso-tracheal suction and even bronchoscopy bronchial secretions are overwhelming or that the patient is becoming exhausted and less co-operative tracheal intubation is necessary. Despite recent enthusiasm for nasotracheal intubation there is little doubt that in treating chest injuries orotracheal tubes are to be preferred. Nasotracheal tubes are inevitably narrower and longer and as they are required to take several bends are more readily obstructed by thick secretions. Furthermore, the introduction of suction catheters through these tubes may be difficult. Although nasotracheal intubation is suitable for infants and children, its use should be avoided in patients with chest injuries or in situations where sputum retention is a problem, cuffed orotracheal tubes being more efficient. With such a tube in place, the patient is enabled to breathe warmed humidified oxygen-enriched air and suction is readily undertaken as often as is necessary. Artificial ventilation may be started at any time.

SUCTION CATHETERS

These should be soft and disposable. Attempts to enter the separate main bronchi by using catheters with rigid, curved ends are traumatic and unsatisfactory. Whereas the right main bronchus is readily entered, there is good evidence that the left is rarely separately entered no matter how ingenious the design of the tube or the manipulation of the operator. The purpose of suction via the endo-tracheal tube is to tickle the sensitive tracheal mucosa producing reflex coughing. Forceful suction with rigid catheters soon damages the tracheal mucosa and depresses the ability of the ciliary action of this mucosa to sweep secretions centrally.

TRACHEOSTOMY

Should the need for tracheal intubation persist, tracheostomy may become necessary. Opinions vary concerning the safe maximum period of orotracheal intubation. Certainly in the days of rubber tubes, laryngeal damage and stricture formation were frequently recorded. Modern tubes of soft plastic are less traumatic and it is safe to leave such tubes in place for up to 1 week or 10 days or even longer before tracheostomy need be considered. When necessary, tracheostomy should be undertaken optimistically and confidently at a time when benefits are possible and should not be reserved for patients in a terminal state. The more frequent use of tracheostomy and widespread understanding of tracheostomy care have made this operation the safe and useful procedure it now is. Tracheostomy and tracheostomy suction are well tolerated by the patient who needs less sedation than the patient with an orotracheal tube.

Operation of Tracheostomy

This should be performed by an experienced surgeon in an operating theatre in good light with adequate surgical assistance and instruments. Although this may be self-evident, one may still encounter the lone doctor attempting tracheostomy in the ward by hand-held lights and with few instruments. That successful tracheostomy is ever completed under these circumstances is cause for congratulation but in no way condones such heroic attempts. The availability of adequate endotracheal tubes has almost completely eliminated the need for emergency tracheostomy and the operation should be delayed until good facilities and competent personnel are available. Should the patient be encumbered by splints, intravenous infusions, chest drainage tubes and various electrical leads, it is quite in order to undertake the operation in the bed rather than move him on to the operating table and this is facilitated in those beds from which the head can be removed.

A small sandbag is placed between the shoulders, enabling the neck to be extended. Local anaesthesia supplemented by minimal doses of inhalation anaesthesia administered via the endotracheal tube is usually adequate.

The skin incision is transverse, 2·5 cm above the suprasternal notch and 5 cm in length. The platysma and pretracheal fascia are opened and the strap muscles held aside by the assistant. It may be necessary to retract or divide the thyroid isthmus. The removal of large discs of trachea or suture of tracheal flaps to the skin are both unnecessary and mutilating and furthermore may be followed by stricture formation at the site of this stoma. An adequate opening into the trachea is readily achieved by a simple longitudinal midline incision through the 2nd, 3rd and perhaps 4th tracheal rings, and when this is held apart an appropriate size tracheostomy tube may be readily introduced. One or two skin sutures on either side of the tube are adequate. The tracheostomy tube tapes should be firmly tied by the surgeon using tight knots with instructions that the tapes be left well alone for 48 hours. Tying these tapes with pretty bows invites well-intentioned staff to interfere with these at the earliest opportunity with possible dislodgement of the tube. After 48 hours the tube may safely be changed.

Care of Tracheostomy

Tracheostomy, while of great benefit to the patient, creates its own acute problems:

1. Increased liability to local and pulmonary infection.
2. Decreased ability of patient to clear his secretions.
3. Inadequate humidification of inspired air.

All procedures involving handling of the tracheostomy should be undertaken using full sterile precautions. The tracheostomy wound should be swabbed with non-irritant antiseptic solutions. Ideally nursing staff should avoid contact with other patients, for cross-infection may become a serious problem in special care units and, when from time to time several patients become infected with organisms such as *Pseudomonas*, *Escherichia coli* or *Staphylococcus*, serious generalized infections may threaten the work of the department. Local infections may not only proceed to tracheal stricture formation but in the short term may cause severe and even fatal pulmonary infection. These patients are often debilitated and septicaemia readily occurs.

As with endotracheal tubes, tracheostomy by-passes the vocal cords interfering with the patient's ability to build up that head of pressure within the lungs, which is necessary to expel secretions. Weak coughing is possible which moves peripheral secretions into the central bronchi but for their further clearance suction is necessary. Furthermore, following the introduction of an endotracheal tube or of a tracheostomy tube it is recognized that within 48 hours the ciliary action of the tracheal mucosa is grossly upset.

Humidification

Humidification is essential, for the nasopharynx which normally provides warming humidification is by-passed. The drying of inspired gases is not only damaging to the tracheal mucosa but encourages thickening of secretions. To ensure adequate humidification it is important that the patient be well hydrated with both oral and intravenous fluids for general tissue dehydration will eventually affect all mucosal surfaces. It may from time to time be useful to inject small quantities of sterile saline down the tracheostomy tube prior to routine suctioning. This certainly aids both coughing and loosening of secretions. It is important, especially in infants, that this is not overdone or considerable amounts of fluid may be absorbed.

Humidifiers, heated or unheated, saturate the inspired air with water vapour, and recently ultrasonic nebulizers which add an extremely fine water spray into the inspired gases have been used with great benefit. (*See also* p. 25.)

The humidifier and connecting tubes should be frequently sterilized.

Care of the Tracheostomy Cuff

The tracheostomy cuff prevents aspiration of nasopharyngeal secretions and forms an airtight fit, enabling the ventilator to build up an appropriate intrabronchial pressure. A well-designed cuff will position the distal end of the tube centrally within the trachea and it is hoped that the inflated cuff exerts minimal pressure on the tracheal mucosa and the tracheal microcirculation. The most suitable form of cuff seems to combine the characteristics of high compliance, softness and large volume, and although numerous types of cuff are in use it is likely that the large volume, floppy cuff will gain wide acceptance.

Grillo et al. (1971) described a tracheostomy tube cuff which is floppy and of large volume which when filled but unstretched is sufficiently large to occlude the trachea. It functions at pressures of the order of one-tenth of those measured in cuffs of standard tracheostomy tubes. This cuff was used in a random series of 45 patients who required tracheostomy for respiratory support. The tracheas of these patients were examined at intervals endoscopically and it was quite clear that the floppy cuff caused little damage and that those patients with severe tracheal ulceration were those in whom standard tracheostomy cuffs had been used (*Fig*. 4). Tracheostomy cuffs may cause other complications which include difficulty of insertion of the tube or of occlusion of the end of the tube if badly fitting.

The ideal tracheostomy tube should be smooth and of inert material, polyvinyl chloride tubing being superior to either metal or rubber. The tube should be non-kinking, the internal diameter remaining constant at body temperature. It should have the largest possible diameter together with the smallest wall thickness commensurate with both strength, flexibility and non-kinking. Although there is a need for a sensitive indicator of cuff pressures these are by no means readily available. With the cuff just inflated to create an airtight seal very little extra air introduced into the cuff is needed to increase pressure on the tracheal wall to a degree which will cause local necrosis, and perhaps late stricture.

Although it might seem obvious that intermittent deflation of the cuff minimizes the risk of ischaemic damage to the tracheal mucosa, such a programme has its disadvantages. In those patients who require ventilation, deflation of the cuff may deprive the tube of its airtight fit and prevent adequate ventilation and allow aspiration of nasopharyngeal secretions. On the other hand, an over-inflated cuff

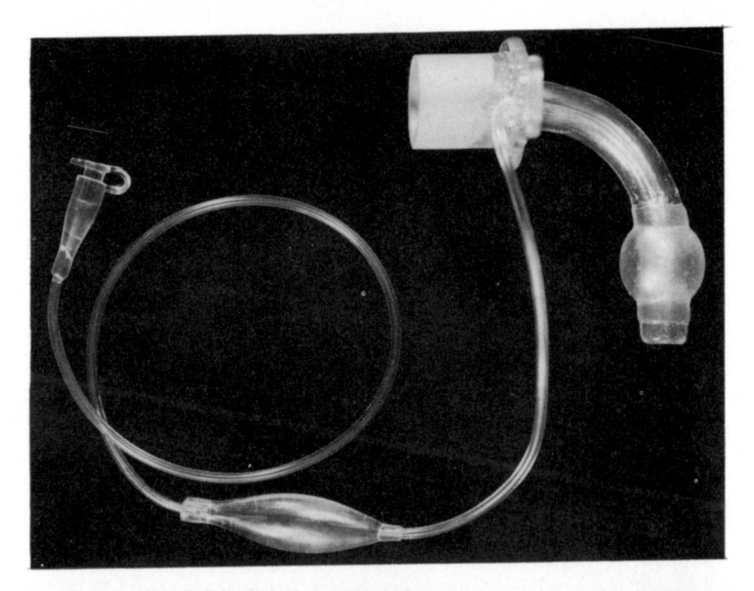

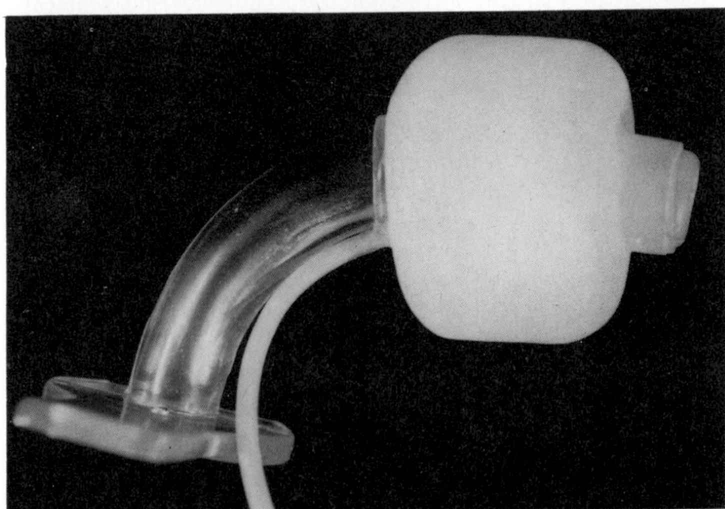

Fig. 4. *Top:* Conventional tracheostomy tube with cuff inflated with 3 ml of air. *Bottom*: Tracheostomy tube carrying latex rubber floppy cuff inflated with 8 ml of air. Pressures measured in the cuffs under these conditions indicate that the floppy cuff pressure is about 10 per cent of that within the standard cuff (Grillo et al., 1971).

will cause ulceration in a very short time, for the tracheal mucosa is soon damaged by pressure necrosis and it is unlikely that any of the currently advised régimes of intermittent inflation and deflation of the cuff will prevent this. It is suggested by some that where possible the cuff should be deflated for 5 minutes in every hour but it is likely that the adoption of low pressure floppy cuffs will prove of greater benefit than such arbitrary periods of cuff deflation.

Post-tracheostomy Strictures

Most reported series of tracheal strictures indicate that the great majority are associated with the use of tracheostomy in the treatment of chest injuries. This may reflect the widespread and perhaps sometimes indiscriminate use of this operation by the less expert in ill-equipped centres, although this complication may follow tracheostomy undertaken with great skill and in a good environment. Apart from clinically manifest tracheal strictures, tracheoscopic and tomographic examination undertaken some months following tracheostomy will in many cases show some degree of tracheal narrowing. Tracheal strictures may complicate tracheostomy or the prolonged use of endotracheal tubes. The stricture may present clinically either shortly after removal of the tracheostomy tube or after a delay of some months. The stricture may be at the site of the inflatable cuff, at the site of the stoma or more distally, when it is due to damage by aspiration catheters. Stomal strictures may be associated with the removal of excessive amounts of tracheal wall at operation or the use of tracheal flaps. The most common aetiological features, however, are pressure necrosis and infection. The adoption of low pressure cuffs and the insistence on aseptic nursing techniques, together with less destructive surgery, should go some way towards reducing the incidence of this complication. A useful review of this subject is provided by Harley (1971).

Removal of Tracheostomy Tube

In due course the tracheostomy tube may be dispensed with. As a primary measure the cuffed tube may be exchanged for a smaller size uncuffed tube, enabling the patient to breathe through the tube and breathe normally. A speaking tube may be used for a time, enabling the patient to cough and speak normally for a trial period, following which the tube may be removed and the wound covered. At this stage it is well worth closing the tracheostomy wound with a few stitches. This will produce a more cosmetic scar.

Mini Tracheostomy

An ingenious device has recently been developed by Matthews that is quite simple in concept. This is the insertion of a 4 or 5 mm internal diameter plastic tube into the trachea via a tiny incision in the crico-thyroid membrane. This tube is readily inserted under local anaesthesia, and provides ready access for suction in patients who are otherwise well able to breathe adequately.

CHOICE OF VENTILATOR

The choice of ventilator depends to some extent on the purpose for which it is to be used, ventilators used during operative surgery perhaps being unsuitable for use in the special care unit. Since ventilators will be largely under the control of junior staff and nurses, it is important that they are simple in construction, easy to handle and have as few snags as is possible with complicated apparatus. Readiness of dismantling, ease of cleaning and sterilization of tubes, ports and valves are important. The controls must be robust and easily handled. The simplest machine which will do all these things is the machine of choice.

It is important to monitor the ventilator to ensure that the metered reading of gas volumes is in fact reaching the patient and several different makes of ventilators are equipped with volume meters.

Volume Cycled Ventilators

These deliver a known volume of gas at a known rate regardless of the state of the airway or of pulmonary compliance or chest wall resistance. Variations in compliance or resistance will be reflected in alterations in the pressure at which the gases are delivered. In an adequately sedated patient with clear airways this pressure remains remarkably constant for that patient and a real increase in delivery pressure, at constant flow rates, might indicate the need for bronchial suction or suggest progressive lung damage. Volume cycled ventilators are particularly useful for the special care unit, are readily understood by the nursing and medical staff, and once mastered may be used with confidence.

Pressure Cycled Ventilators

These deliver a flow of gas which is cut off when a predetermined pressure is attained. Even in experienced hands such ventilators are prone to temperamental behaviour and thus are often of less value for long term ventilation. They have, however, the advantage of 'patient triggering'. Patients requiring long term ventilation need this to be controlled but following long term ventilation dependence on the machine is common and may defy efforts to wean the patient to spontaneous and effective breathing. In such patients short periods using a triggered respirator may help develop confidence, the patient entering a half-way house of self-triggering which may be a short step to independence.

Pressure cycled machines such as the Bird and Bennett ventilators are well known and are reliable when used by experts.

Some ventilators combine the features of both pressure and volume cycled mechanisms but these tend to be complicated and may confuse junior medical and nursing staff.

CONTINUOUS POSITIVE AIRWAY PRESSURE (CPAP) BREATHING WITH SPONTANEOUS VENTILATION IN THE MANAGEMENT OF CHEST INJURIES

CPAP, otherwise 'continuous positive end expiratory pressure', has been used successfully in the treatment of the respiratory distress syndrome of the newborn and in cardiac surgery. As the name implies, this technique involves positive airway pressure at the end of expiration and throughout the expiratory phase of the respiratory cycle, the degree of positive pressure being adjusted by the level of an underwater seal, or by a special valve. The effect of CPAP is often predictable and is not always beneficial, for continuous positive pressure within the thorax will impede venous return in many patients. However, in most patients its use is associated with improvement of respiratory efficiency and an increase in arterial oxygen tension.

An important indication for CPAP is the period following continuous positive pressure ventilation during which the patient may still to some extent be dependant on support by the ventilator. In these patients weaning from the ventilator dependence to normal spontaneous breathing is often considerably facilitated. A more recent use of CPAP has been in the management of patients with severe chest injuries whose own respiratory efforts may be inadequate. The addition of 5–10 cm of CPAP has been shown to help these patients considerably.

Humidifiers

Ventilators should include a humidifier in the inspiratory limb capable of producing full or super humidification to ensure that secretions are kept at a low viscosity and that the respiratory mucous membrane is not allowed to dry. Humidifiers are unfortunately particularly liable to contamination with pathogenic organisms and must therefore be readily detachable for sterilization. Bacterial cross-infection is an ever-present hazard in special care units and the use of bacterial filters is now recognized as an important prophylactic measure.

Unfortunately, the 'universal ventilator' suited to all situations and patients is an illusion and it is usual to rely on perhaps two main types for use in the special care unit.

Intermittent Mandatory Ventilation (IMV)

The technique of reducing the frequency of respiratory cycles of the ventilator in a gradual fashion, and allowing the patient to breathe spontaneously for part of the time, is a valuable method of weaning patients from the ventilator.

Chapter 5

Radiological features of chest injuries

Chest radiographs of good quality and repeated frequently are necessary for the accurate diagnosis and effective treatment of the patient with a chest injury. Unhappily, chest radiography is under-used often with serious consequences. All patients who have been involved in a road traffic accident or a fall from a height deserve a chest radiograph. It is frequently maintained that some are so severely injured that chest radiography might be dangerous, but there can be few situations where a patient is too ill for this to be done. It must be borne in mind that the cause of the patient's serious state may in fact be haemothorax or pneumothorax and if un-diagnosed and untreated no improvement is to be expected.

With the exception of critically ill patients chest radiography should be conducted with the patient sitting upright. Should this procedure be unduly prolonged the patient may become distressed. Such delays occur while the radiographer, having made the patient sit up and having positioned the X-ray film, searches for a suitable electric socket, changes the tube distance or begins to estimate the appropriate exposure time. All should be made ready with the machine plugged in and switched on and these calculations predeter-mined. With the radiographer's finger on the button, two suitably protected persons should sit the patient up, place an X-ray plate behind the chest and expose the film. With care this should occupy no more than 10 or 15 seconds. The radiograph so obtained may be of great value.

Chest radiographs exposed with the patient lying flat are often deceptive. A collection of both blood and air in the pleural cavity forms a three-layered sandwich of air, lung and blood. The radiodense blood and the radiotranslucent air tend to cancel each other out and a casual glance at such a chest radiograph might arouse little comment (*Fig.* 5). A patient with a radiograph exposed 5 minutes later while sitting upright might have a large haemopneumothorax (*Figs.* 6–8). Chest radiography should be repeated once or twice daily and should be repeated after chest aspiration or operation. Following an apparently minor injury the chest radiograph may appear normal. However, from time to time pneumothorax or haemothorax may develop a day or two later presumably due to damage by rib fragments. Such a patient reported after a fall and was shown to have a fractured right clavicle. Two days later dyspnoea prompted further radiography which showed (*Fig.* 9) the previously expanded lung to be collapsed by pneumothorax. Rib fractures are not always noted, as they are obscured by chest wall contusions, lung contusions, haemothorax or surgical emphysema. Some fractures become radiologically demonstrable only after some weeks with the tell-tale development of callus. The lateral film may demonstrate some rib fractures more clearly and indicate a fractured sternum.

The size of pneumothorax is important and any suggestion of a tension situation will stimulate urgent tube drainage. Haemothorax is evident and a fluid level in the pleura confirms the presence of air and fluid in the pleural cavity.

Radiographic evidence of bowel in the chest will indicate traumatic rupture of the diaphragm, more commonly noted on the left side (*Fig.* 10).

Close attention should be paid to the size of the upper mediastinal shadow and a suggestion of widening should arouse suspicion of traumatic rupture of the aorta (*Fig.* 11). Subcutaneous or mediastinal emphysema is readily visible in the radiograph and usually confirms the known clinical feature (*Fig.* 12). However, mediastinal emphysema may be detected radiologically long before it spreads to the neck and should suggest possible lung or oesophageal injury.

In the course of an accident foreign bodies may enter the chest and be noted radiologically. The commonest are gunshot but from time to time the patient may inhale a broken tooth or his own dental plate. Unfortunately, the plastic material of dental plates is usually radiotranslucent.

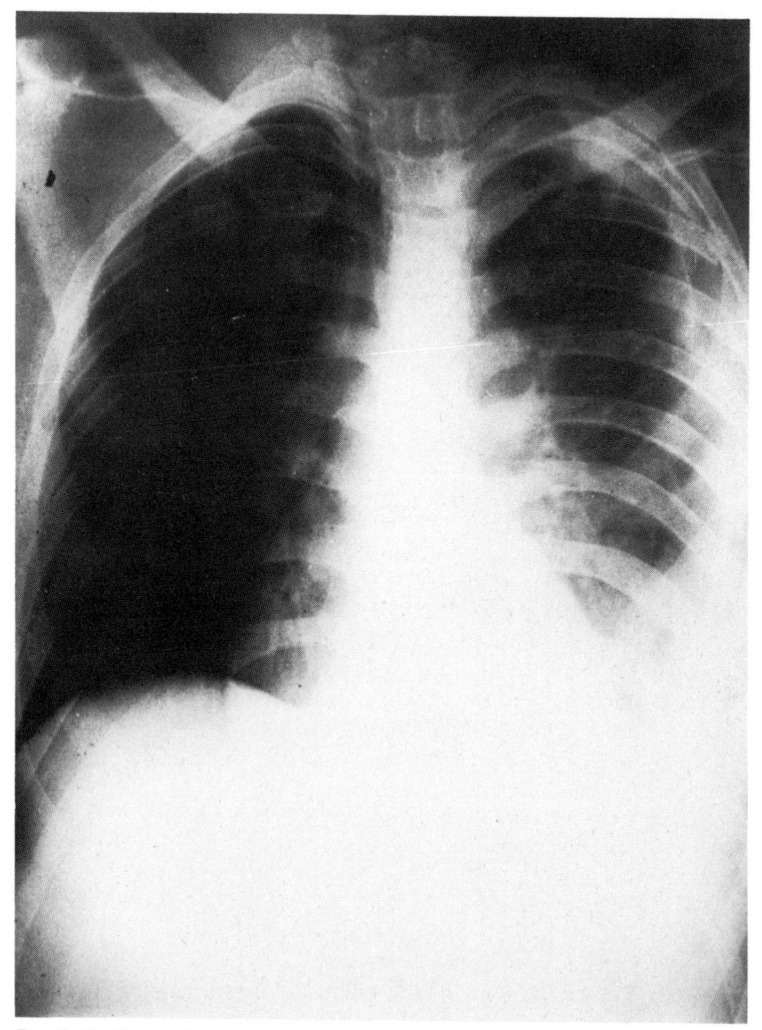

Fig. 5. Radiograph taken with patient lying flat following chest injury. This demonstrates a small pneumothorax with some fluid at the base.

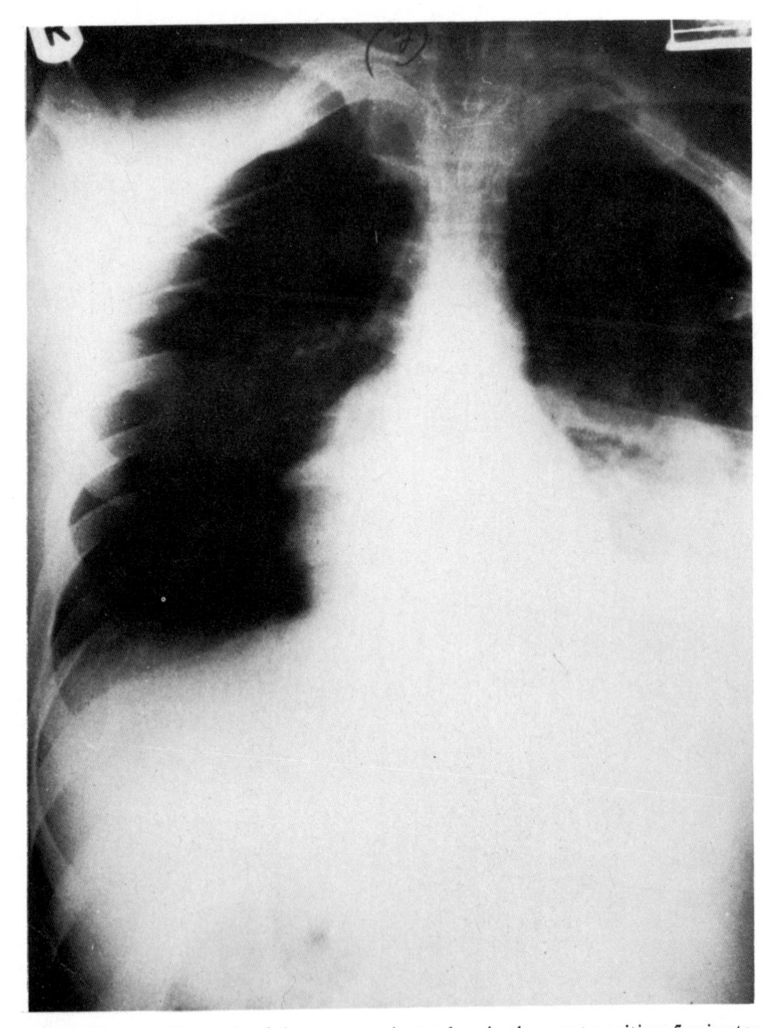

Fig. 6. Chest radiograph of the same patient taken in the erect position 5 minutes after *Fig*. 5 was taken. A large pneumothorax is now apparent and 1·5 litres of blood were removed following intercostal drainage.

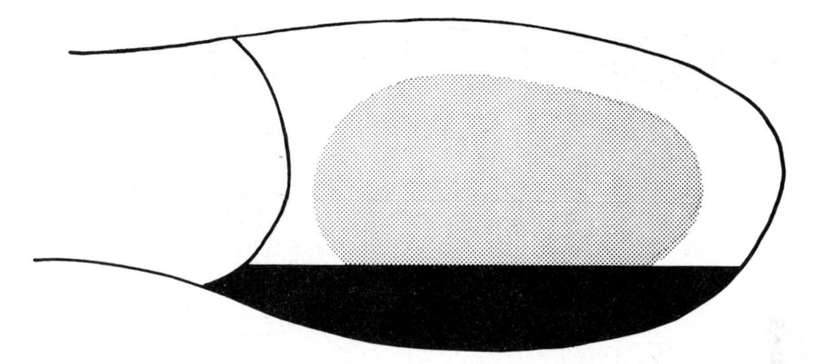

Fig. 7. Diagrammatic representation of the three-layered sandwich of air, lung and blood which appears in the supine position and which may cause confusion radiologically.

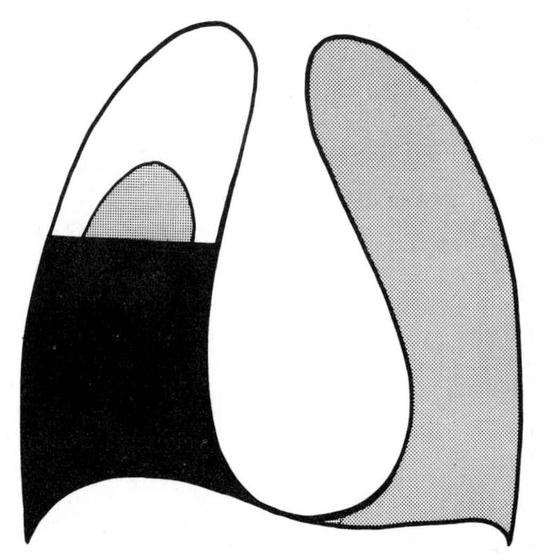

Fig. 8. When taken in the erect position the effusion, pneumothorax and lung tend to be more readily identified radiologically.

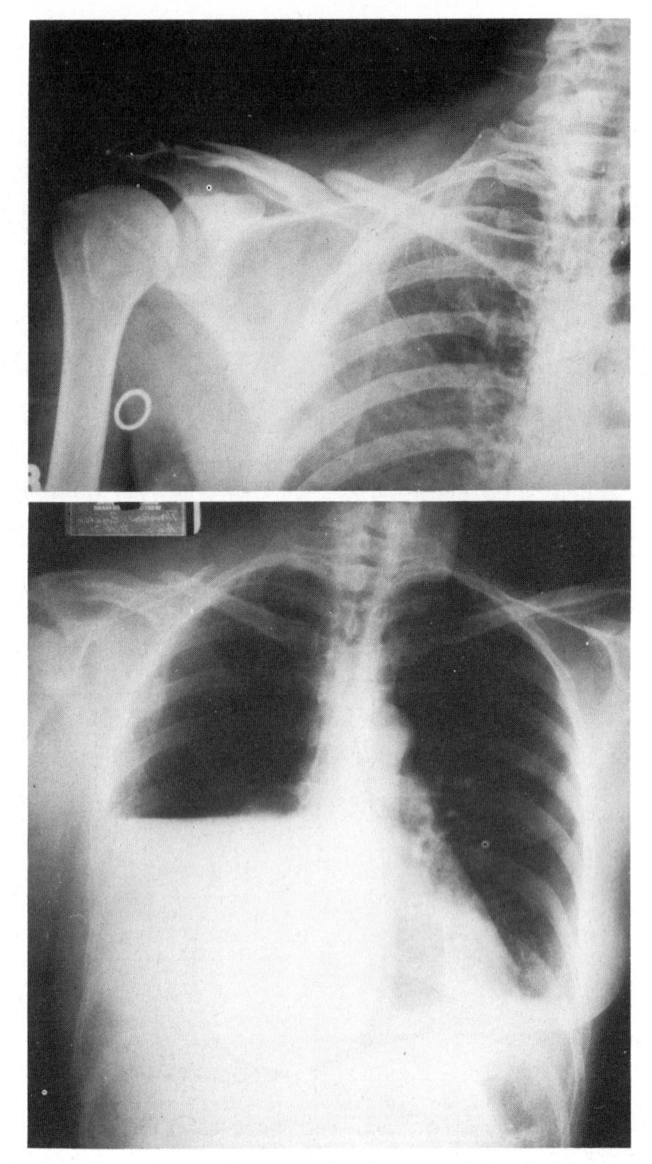

Fig. 9. A radiograph (*top*) demonstrating fracture of the clavicle showed no evidence of pneumothorax, but the radiograph taken 2 days following injury when the patient complained of shortness of breath clearly demonstrates a large haemopneumothorax.

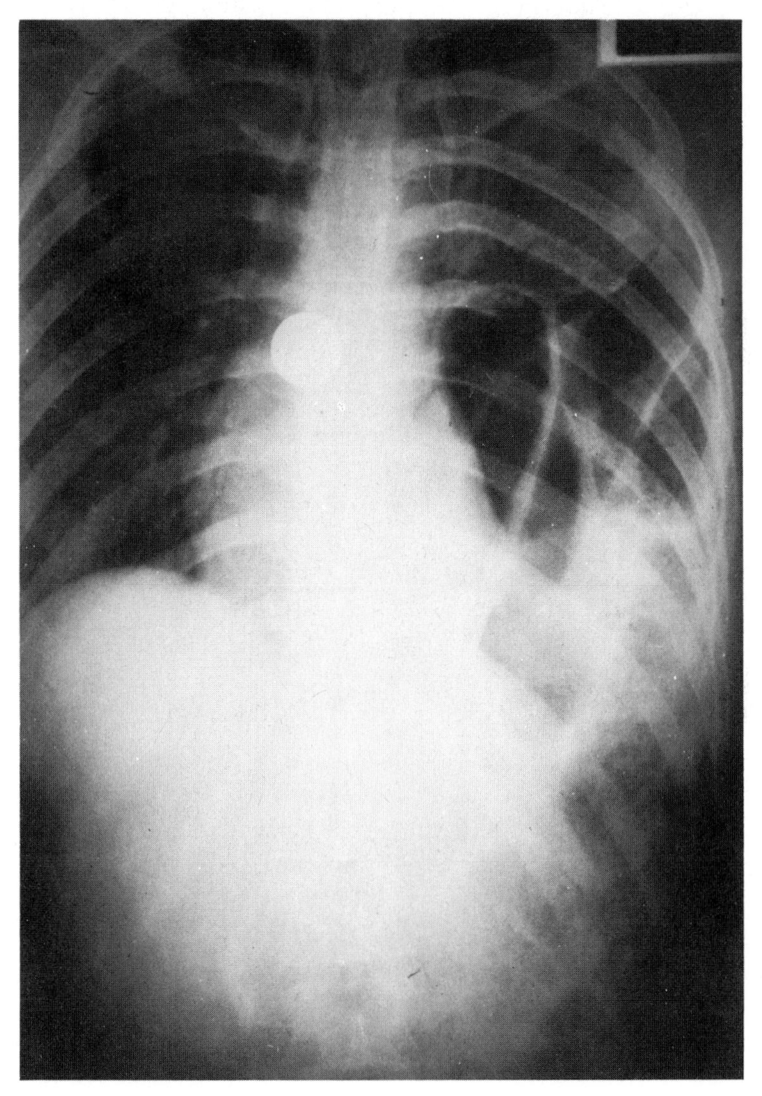

Fig. 10. Traumatic rupture of the left diaphragm.

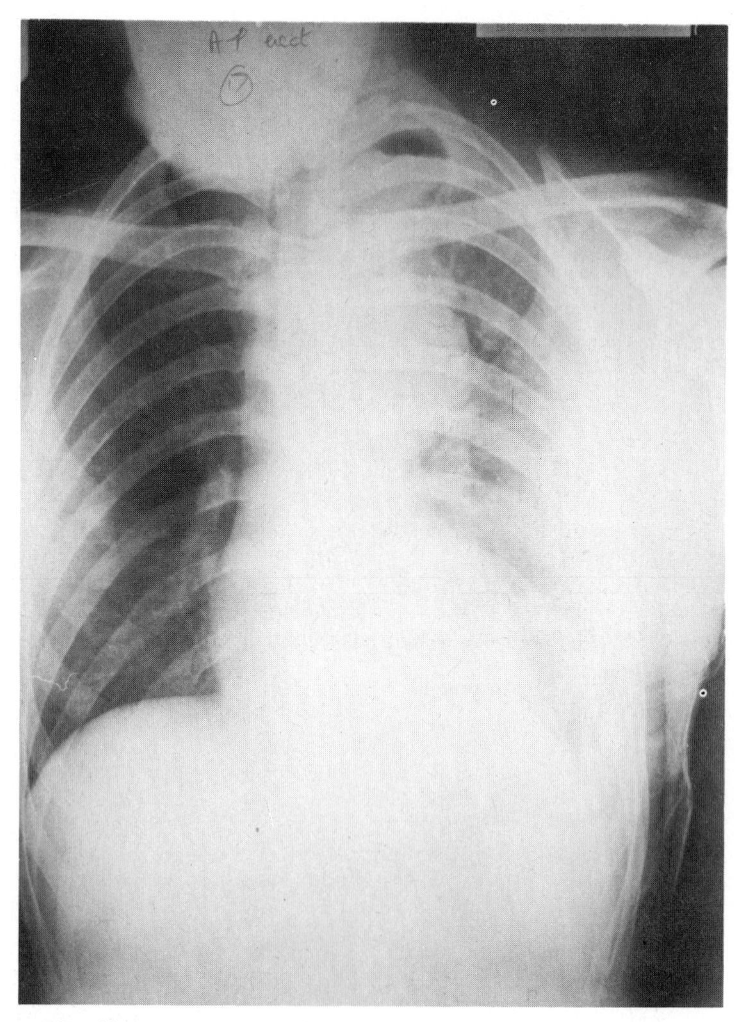

Fig. 11. Traumatic mediastinal haematoma following a car accident.

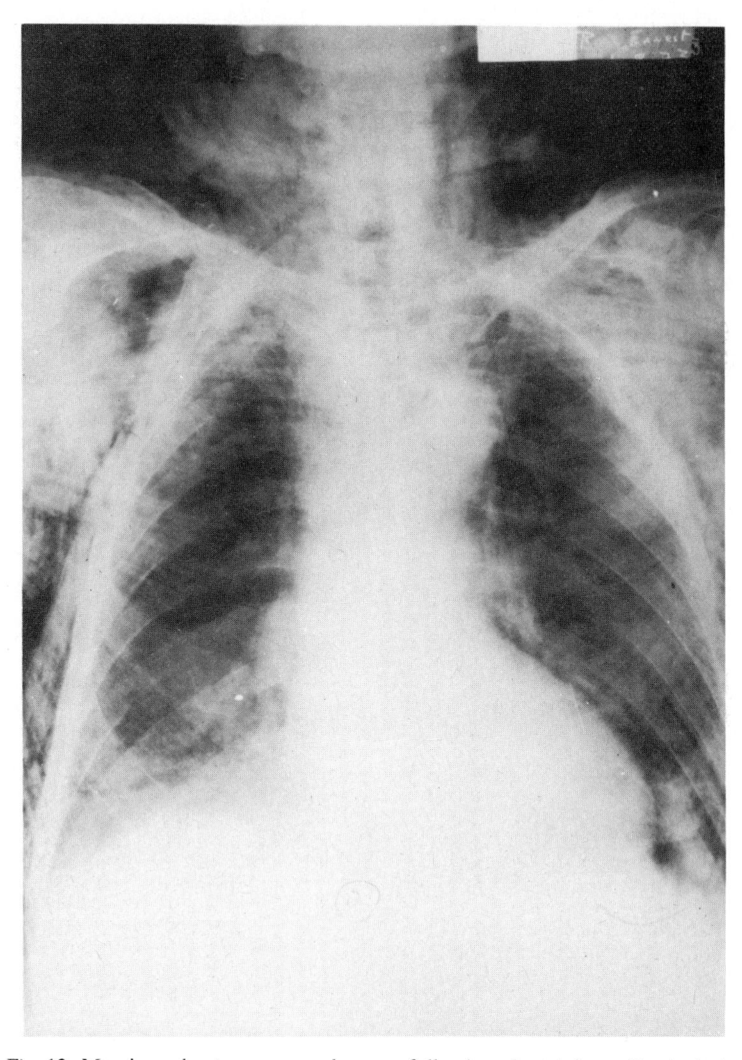

Fig. 12. Massive subcutaneous emphysema following chest injury. Particularly well shown is the fan-like appearance of the pectoralis major muscles so characteristic of this condition.

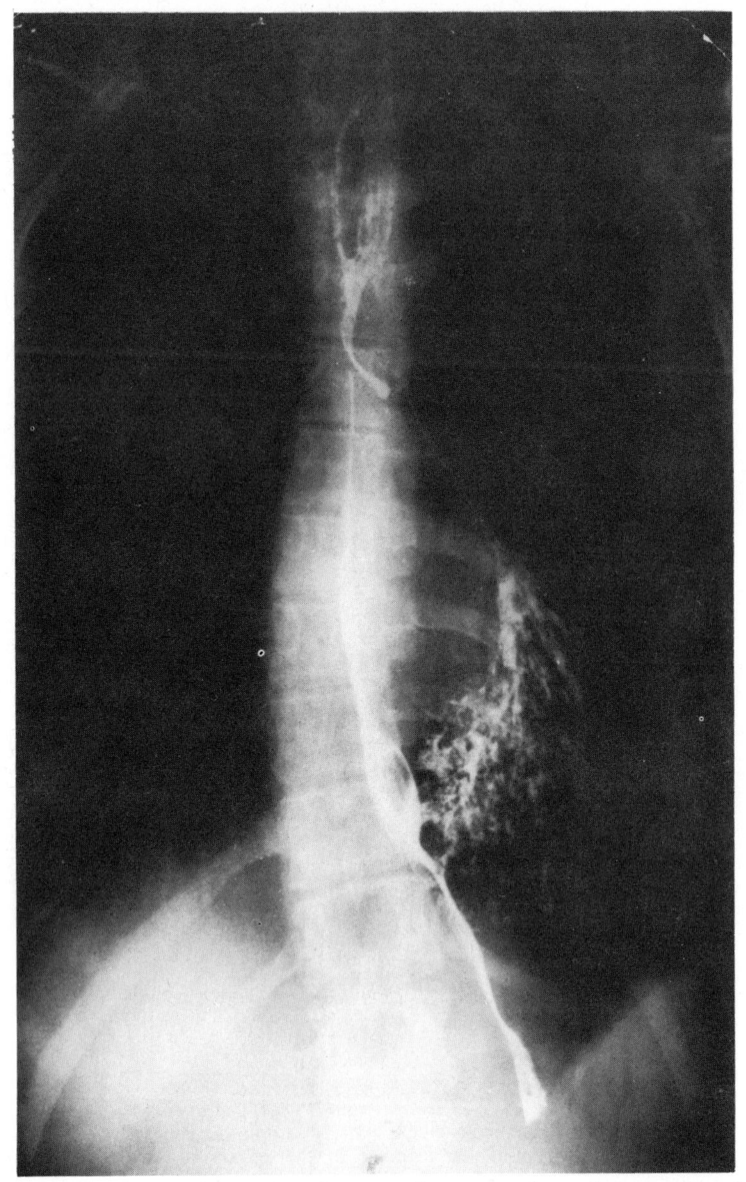

Fig. 13*a*. Gastrografin swallow demonstrating traumatic tracheo-oesophageal fistula following a car accident. (*See Fig.* 16.)

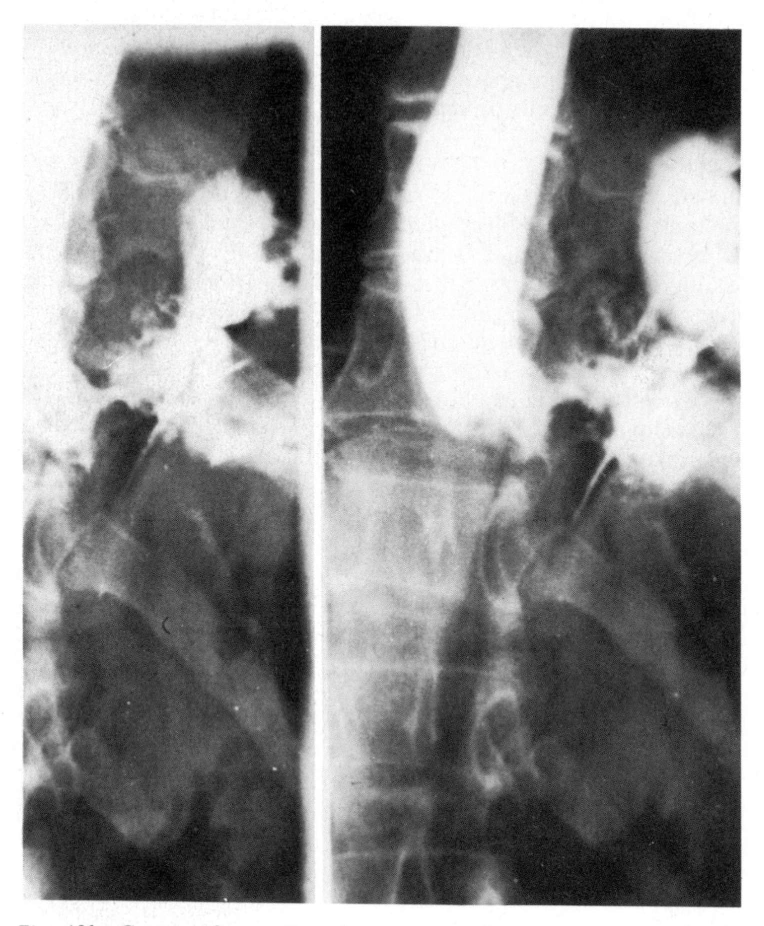

Fig. 13*b*. Gastrografin swallow demonstrating instrumental perforation of oesophagus.

OTHER RADIOLOGICAL INVESTIGATIONS

Contrast Radiography

Suspicion of damage to the oesophagus is best investigated by Gastrografin swallow. From time to time contrast radiography of the bronchial tree may assist in the diagnosis of bronchial strictures secondary to previous trauma (*Fig.* 13*a*, *b*).

Angiocardiography

Should damage to the great vessels be suspected, aortography is recommended. This investigation is readily undertaken in many X-ray departments and is best carried out by the percutaneous Seldinger method using either the femoral artery or the brachial artery. The tip of the catheter is positioned 5 cm above the aortic valve prior to automatic pressure injection of contrast material. Multiple consecutive radiographs (4 per second) are usually of greater value than cineradiography in these circumstances (*Fig.* 14).

Occasionally cardiac catheterization and angiocardiography are undertaken to help diagnose possible traumatic damage to valves and cardiac septa.

CT Scanning

The indications for using computerized tomography (CT) scanning in the assessment of chest injuries are not clear and there is little information that would indicate any advantage over conventional radiology.

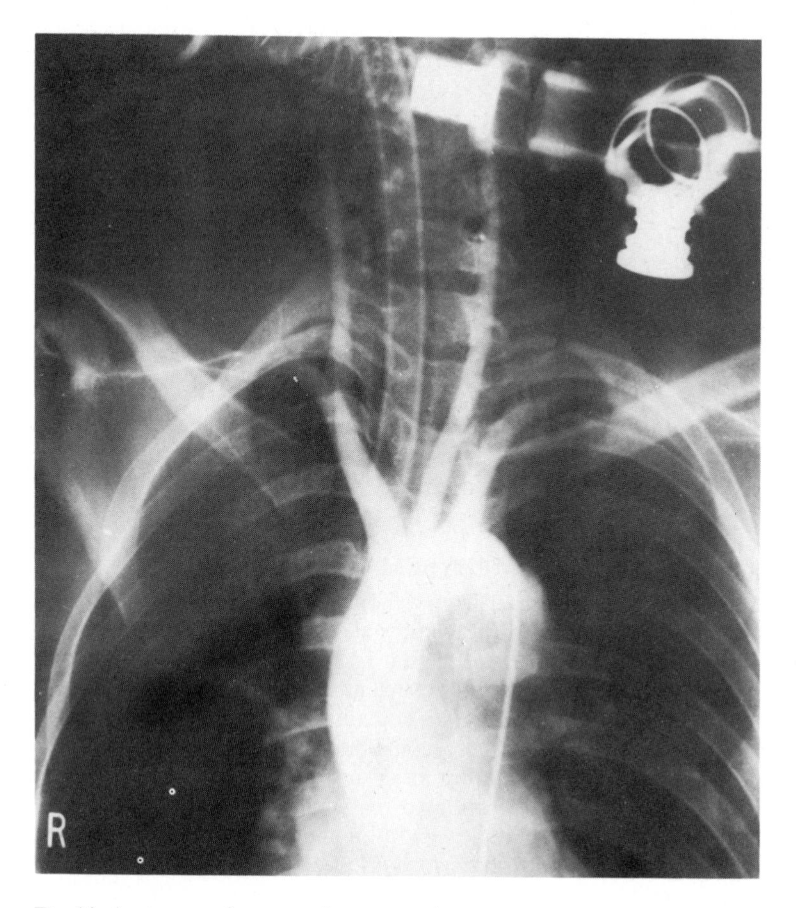

Fig. 14. Aortogram demonstrating traumatic rupture of aorta (patient demonstrated in *Fig*. 11).

Chapter 6

Traumatic emphysema

Following injuries to the chest, air may escape from the respiratory passages or oesophagus and find its way into the subcutaneous tissues or into the mediastinum.

SUBCUTANEOUS EMPHYSEMA (*see Fig.* 12)
This follows escape of air from a damaged lung or air passage which then finds its way into the chest wall and subcutaneous tissues by way of a tear in the parietal pleura. It is occasionally associated with an open chest wound, when external air finds its way into the tissues. Its speed of accumulation gives some indication of the degree of air leak and those patients who become blown up very rapidly should be suspected of having rupture of a main bronchus. Subcutaneous emphysema is often associated with a partially or completely obliterated pleura or with severe pulmonary emphysema, collapse of the lung with pneumothorax formation occurring less readily under these conditions. A large pneumothorax associated with subcutaneous emphysema implies a large air leak. The emphysema occasionally spreads rapidly to involve the entire chest wall and abdomen, sometimes with massive enlargement of the scrotum and may extend to the feet, neck and face as high as the insertion of the scalp aponeurosis. The appearance of the patient may become grotesque, being blown up to resemble a snowman and the eyelids may close (*Fig.* 15). All patients with extreme forms of this condition look alike and it may be some days before they are recognizable by their relatives.

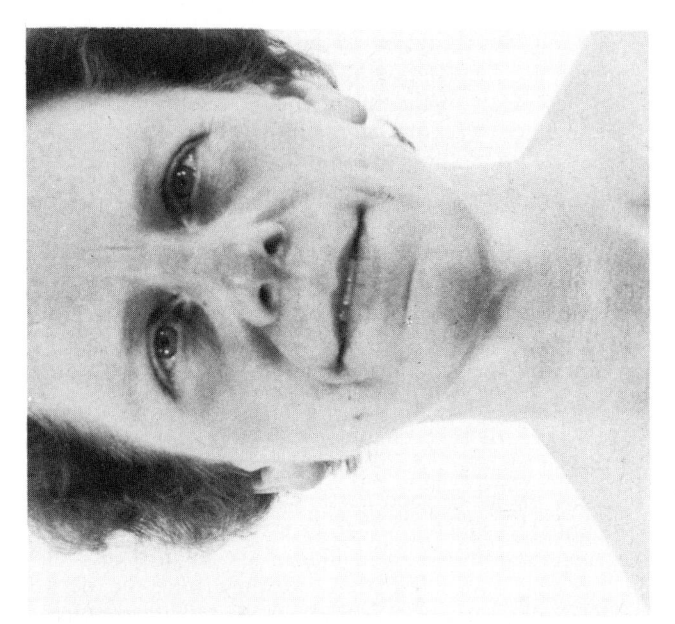

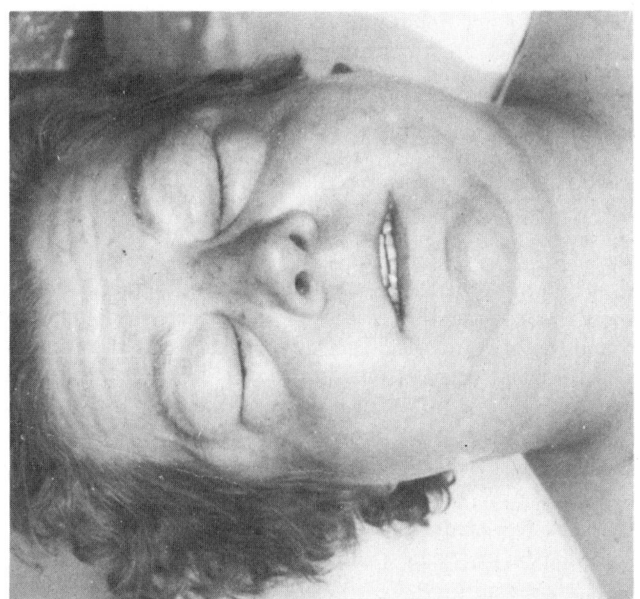

Fig. 15. *Left*: Severe subcutaneous emphysema following chest injury. *Right*: Same patient following subsidence of emphysema.

Despite the terrifying appearance this condition produces few serious symptoms, the condition of the patient relating more to the underlying injuries. Chest radiographs are characteristic, demonstrating the presence of air in the subcutaneous tissues and the fascial planes. The presence of air among the muscle fibres of the pectoralis major muscles clearly outlines their fan-like appearance.

Treatment

Usually no specific treatment is required, as attention is concentrated on treatment of the underlying cause and resolution is usually rapid. The emphysema will increase further with violent coughing and if this persists it may be necessary to pass an endotracheal tube, as this manœuvre prevents the build up of high intrathoracic pressure.

MEDIASTINAL EMPHYSEMA (*Fig.* 16)

The presence of mediastinal emphysema implies a breach of continuity of either the air or food passages within the chest. This may follow lung injury in which alveolar air escapes and dissects into the vascular structures towards the hilum of the lung, thence up and down the mediastinum, ultimately escaping into the neck and becoming clinically obvious. Mediastinal air readily ruptures into the pleura, producing pneumothorax which may become bilateral and consequently dangerous. Should mediastinal air be unable to escape, the increased mediastinal pressure may rarely cause obstruction of the trachea and great veins. When associated with oesophageal lacerations mediastinal emphysema assumes serious significance for a rapidly spreading cellulitis and mediastinitis may follow.

Diagnosis

Mediastinal air may be noted on the chest radiograph and occur with subcutaneous crackling in the neck. Retrosternal pain may be present and a hoarse voice is characteristic. Apart from chest injuries mediastinal emphysema may occur after severe coughing, after recent endoscopic procedures or as a result of positive pressure ventilation.

Treatment

The treatment for mediastinal emphysema is to treat the cause. Thus, oesophageal or tracheal rupture requires surgical closure. The majority of patients, however, have no serious underlying injury and resolution is usually spontaneous and not long delayed. Very rarely,

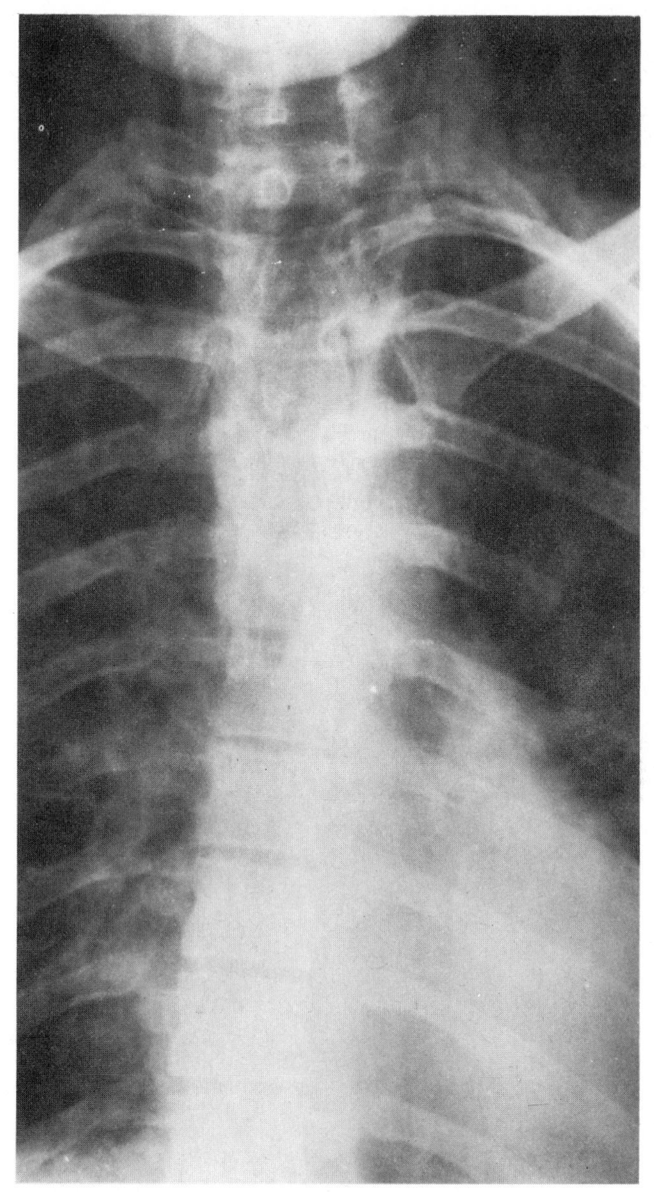

Fig. 16. Mediastinal emphysema following car accident which caused traumatic rupture of the oesophagus. (*See Fig*. 13*a*.)

cervical mediastinostomy is necessary in order to decompress the abnormally distended mediastinum.

Under local anaesthesia a 5-cm transverse incision is made just above the suprasternal notch and after division of the pretracheal fascia a finger is introduced into the mediastinum in the plane of the trachea much as in the operation of mediastinoscopy. This blunt dissection is rewarded by a rush of air and the wound should be kept open by soft latex drains for a few days followed by delayed primary suture.

Chapter 7

Traumatic pneumothorax and haemothorax

Pneumothorax following closed chest injury is usually associated with damage to the lung or air passages, although rarely, closed traumatic rupture of the oesophagus may be responsible. The pneumothorax may be small or large, unilateral or bilateral, and especially in children rib fractures are not necessarily present.

Associated injuries are common and may divert attention from the chest, delaying diagnosis of a potentially lethal condition. This is particularly so with head injuries where loss of consciousness precludes complaints of pain or shortness of breath. The physical signs of pneumothorax may be present but are sometimes difficult to elicit, especially in those with multiple injuries. There is no substitute for radiography (*Fig.* 17).

Although the distinction between simple pneumothorax and tension pneumothorax is acknowledged, it is perhaps useful to appreciate that the merging of one with the other is indistinct, and that simple pneumothorax may develop into a dangerous tension situation with little or no warning (*Figs.* 18 and 19).

A small amount of air in the pleural space will produce few or no symptoms and be readily absorbed. A large collection may cause anoxia due to loss of lung function, although surprisingly total pneumothorax may on occasion produce few symptoms. With the development of tension pneumothorax, in addition to collapse of the lung on the injured side, the mediastinum will be pushed across and the contralateral or 'good' lung will suffer compression collapse. There is no evidence to support the commonly held view that the serious symptoms of this condition are due to mediastinal shift. Anoxia alone is responsible.

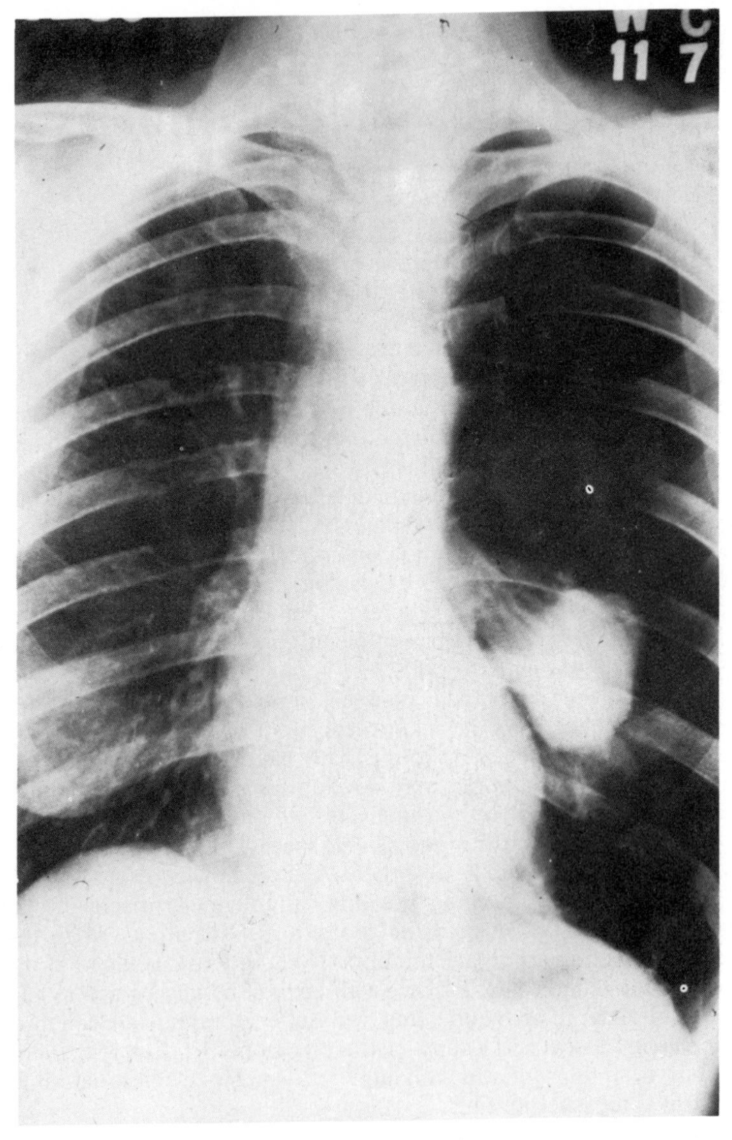

Fig. 17. Traumatic pneumothorax.

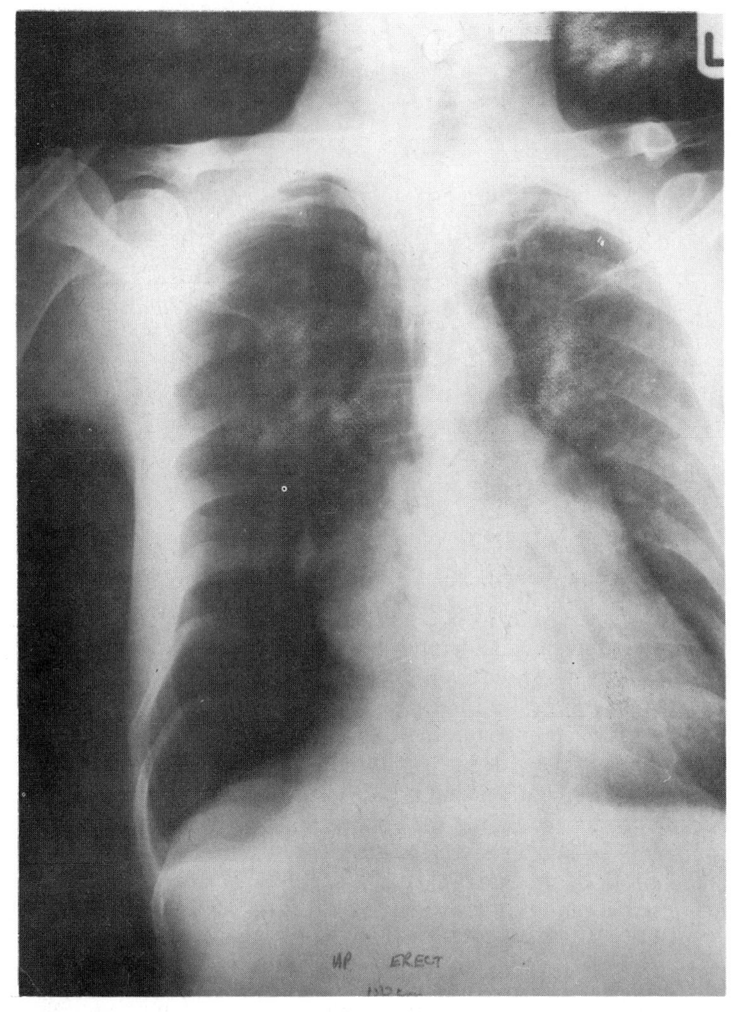

Fig. 18. Traumatic right tension pneumothorax. The heart and mediastinum are displaced towards the left and the right diaphragm is pushed downwards.

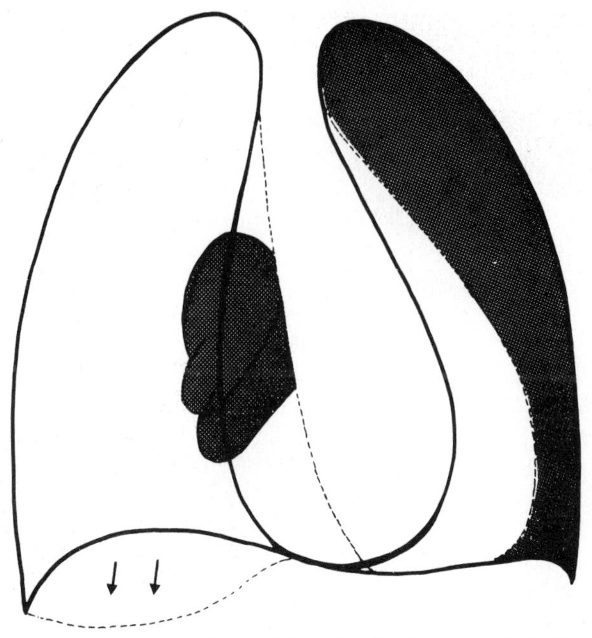

Fig. 19. Right tension pneumothorax. Note the displacement of the heart and mediastinum away from the injury with depression of the diaphragm.

Rarely, mediastinal emphysema caused by oesophageal or bronchial rupture may produce high mediastinal pressures but fortunately the mediastinal pleura offers little support with consequent rupture and pneumothorax.

A greater or less degree of bleeding into the pleural space may accompany traumatic pneumothorax, with both blood loss and space-occupying clot increasing the anoxia. Furthermore, associated lung contusions or flail chest may aggravate the condition. Evacuation of pneumothorax is readily achieved and will help the patient to tolerate other injuries and facilitate anaesthesia.

TENSION PNEUMOTHORAX

When the pleural surface of the lung is torn in such a manner that it acts as a one-way valve, air will escape into the pleural cavity with each breath, and as this progresses a tension situation develops with mediastinal shift and compression collapse of the other lung. This may happen to patients with lacerated lung surfaces who require treatment by intermittent positive pressure ventilation and in whom

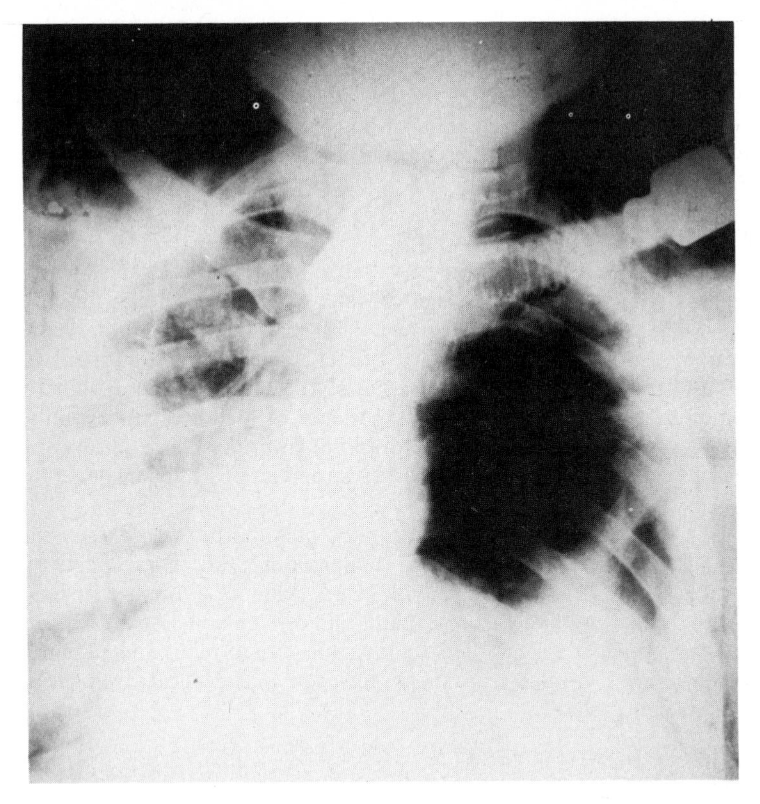

Fig. 20. Left tension pneumothorax associated with positive pressure ventilation. It is likely that air was forced into the pleural cavity through the damaged lung surface.

the ventilator pressure readily forces air into the pleural space with consequent tension pneumothorax (*Fig.* 20).

Treatment

In an emergency tension pneumothorax may be relieved by the insertion of a wide-bored needle into the pleural space, rewarded by a rush of escaping air and corresponding improvement in the patient's condition. It is, however, emphasized that such treatment should be avoided unless the situation is urgent, for in the absence of radiological confirmation of the diagnosis serious mischief can be done.

Other than in an emergency there is little place for needle aspiration of traumatic pneumothorax. Although rapid expansion of the lung may be achieved, the nature of the underlying injury often determines the inevitable redevelopment of pneumothorax, and this may occur many hours later. The practice of attaching an intrapleural wide-bored needle to a tube leading to an underwater seal is mentioned only to be condemned. The needle point soon impinges on the re-expanding lung causing further damage. This misguided practice is, however, beloved by those with little knowledge of the management of the pleural space.

There has recently become available the Heimlich valve, which when attached to an intercostal catheter allows air to leave, but not to re-enter the chest, dispensing with the need for underwater drainage. Although such valves are effective in the treatment of spontaneous pneumothorax, they are to be avoided in traumatic pneumothorax. The author has experience of such a valve becoming jammed with coagulated blood draining from the chest, allowing a simple pneumothorax to deteriorate into a serious tension pneumothorax.

The treatment of choice in traumatic pneumothorax is intercostal catheter drainage connected to underwater seal. This effectively removes air and blood and provides clear evidence of further air leak. The lung is more likely to re-expand and remain so using a catheter; the surgeon is then enabled to turn his attention to the patient's other injuries confident in the knowledge that pleural drainage is effective and reliable.

TECHNIQUE OF INSERTION OF INTERCOSTAL CATHETER

Site

Although some recommend that intercostal catheters be inserted in the midaxillary line, this may lead to difficulties, especially in inexperienced hands. In this position the ribs are close together and the intercostal spaces are narrow. With obese patients the catheter frequently fails to penetrate the chest wall and then lies deep in the axillary fat.

The safest, easiest and most reliable site is the second intercostal space anteriorly in the midclavicular line. A very recent radiograph must confirm the presence of an air space and, if this precaution is never ignored, damage to either the lung or other structures is avoided. Penetrating the chest too close to the sternum might damage the internal mammary vessels, superior vena cava or ascending aorta, so this operation should not be left to an unsupervised beginner. It is well to be certain that the space to be entered is a pleural space and not a large air cyst of the lung, or a herniated

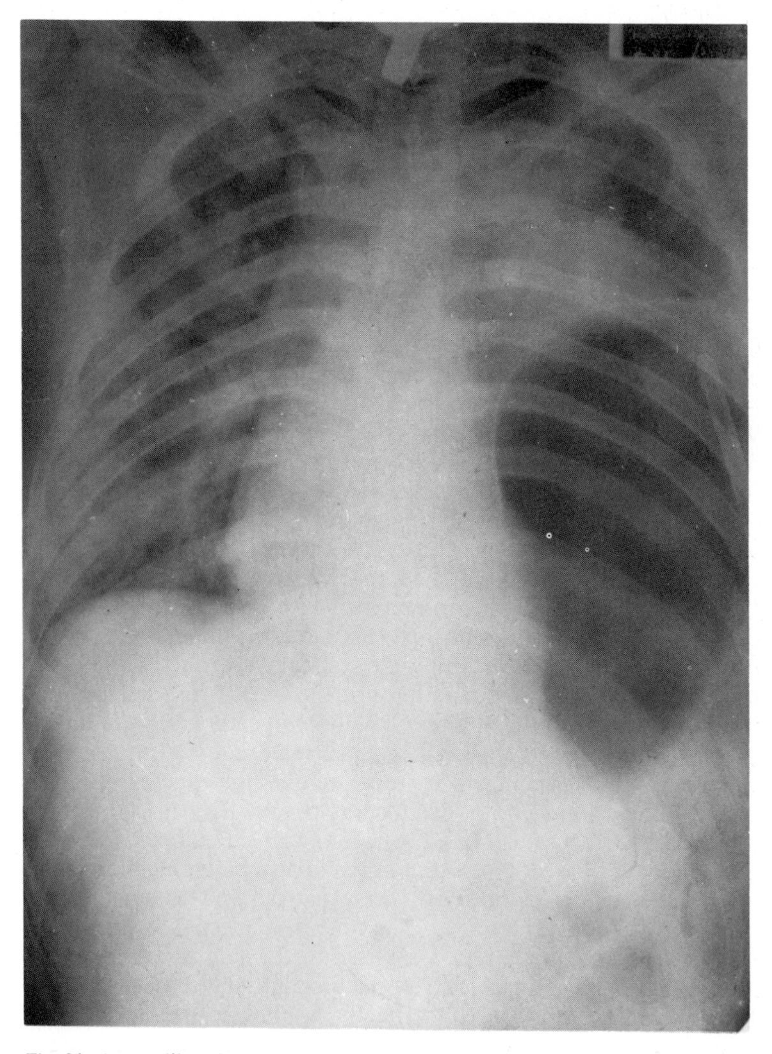

Fig. 21. Acute dilatation of the stomach following chest injury. Intercostal tube drainage of this organ was undertaken following a diagnosis of tension pneumothorax.

intrathoracic stomach. The author has experience of intercostal drainage of both of these structures with less than gratifying results (*Fig.* 21).

Method

Instruments required (*Fig.* 22):

Syringes, needles and local anaesthetic solution
Pointed scalpel blade
Two needles and sutures
Needle holder and artery forceps
Two sizes of trocar and cannula
Catheters and introducer
Sterile tubing
Underwater seal bottle

The tube is best inserted with the patient sitting upright at 60°, ensuring that the underlying lung falls away from the chest wall (*Fig.* 23). The patient's head should be turned away. A subcutaneous weal is raised with local anaesthesia at the site of insertion, and all layers of the chest wall are infiltrated with local anaesthesia. It is important to introduce the needle into the chest cavity to ensure that an air space has been entered. A 1-cm incision is made with a pointed scalpel into the anaesthetized area. A suture is then passed across the incision, its ends loosely tied, and will remain in position until the tube is withdrawn when it may be tied, sealing the incision. The catheter of choice is examined to ensure that it will pass through the cannula, for it is disconcerting to find that the only catheter on the trolley is too large to pass through the already-inserted cannula. The trocar and cannula are then boldly but gently inserted into the pleural space and the trocar is then removed. This movement usually causes coughing. The tube on the introducer is passed through the cannula into the pleural cavity. The trocar is then removed over the tube. The advantage of using a catheter such as a Malecot or De Pezzer type is that it requires only the functional part of the tube to be in the chest, the expanded end to some extent preventing accidental removal. The tube is connected to the underwater seal. A second suture is inserted in the skin and tied several times around the point of entry of the tube into the chest, and a firm dressing applied. It is as well to attach the tubing to the patient's bed by a safety pin, but this connection should be undone when moving the patient or making the bed. In the absence of suitable trocars and cannulae, a tube may be introduced into the pleural cavity by blunt dissection with an artery forceps. Although crude, this method is effective.

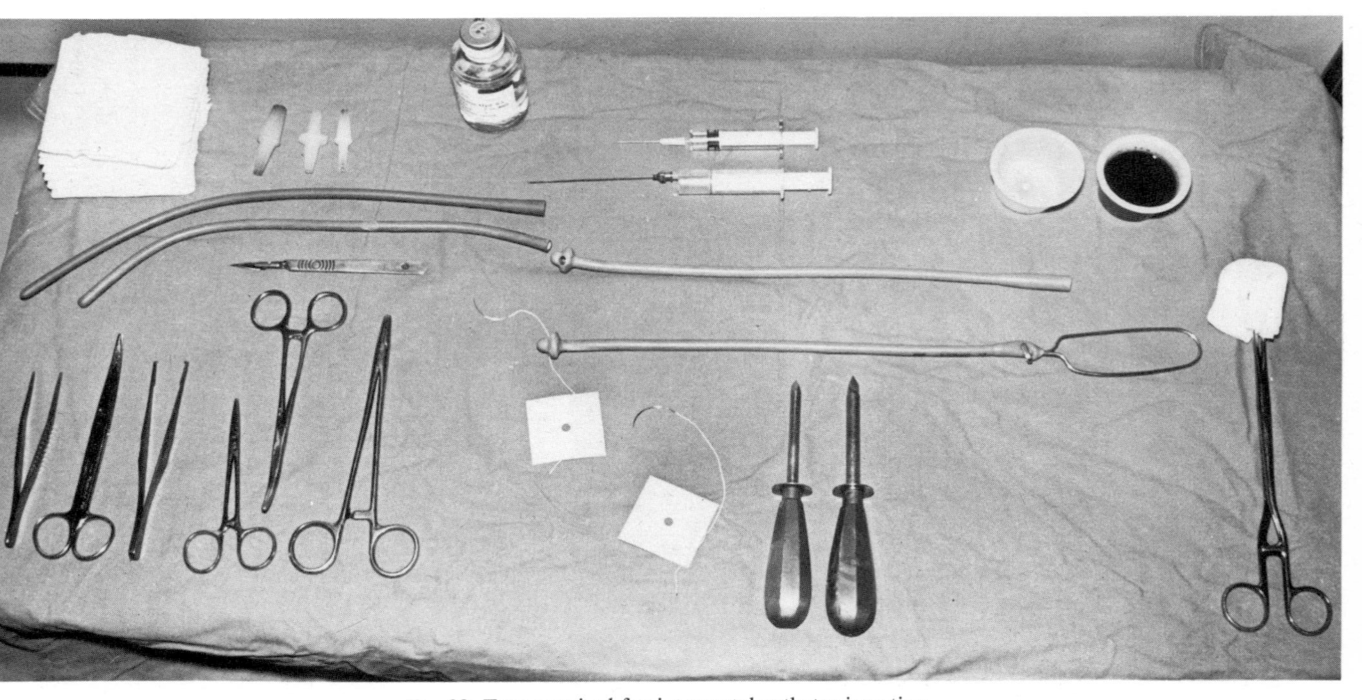

Fig. 22. Tray required for intercostal catheter insertion.

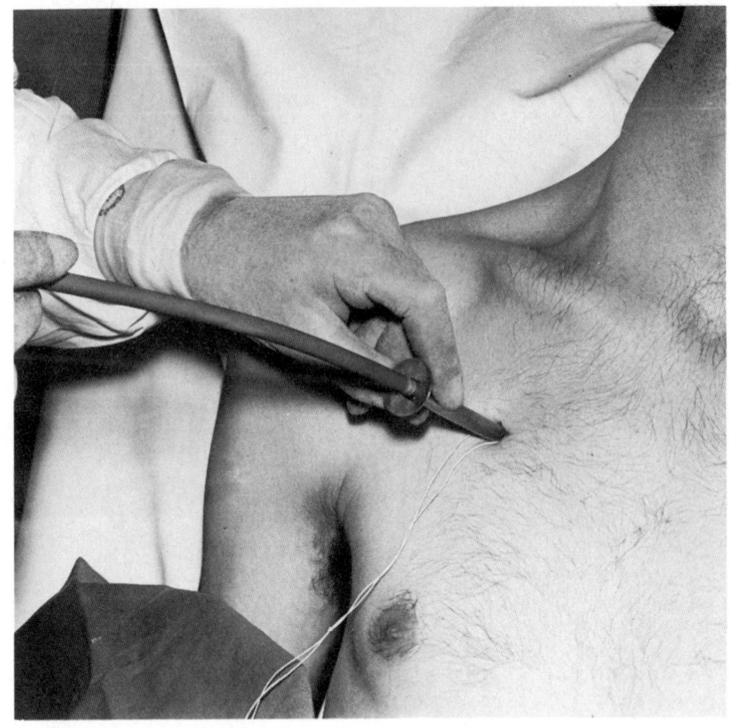

Fig. 23. Insertion of intercostal catheter into the second intercostal space anteriorly in the midclavicular line.

UNDERWATER SEAL (*Fig*. 24)

Although the principle of the underwater seal seems well understood, from time to time serious accidents arise following mishandling of this apparatus by inexperienced or untrained staff. A large stable bottle should be used, for tall narrow bottles, unless held in a special device, are easily knocked over. There should be at least 7 cm of water in the bottle and the catheter from the chest must be connected to the tube which leads 4 cm under water. There must be an extra hole in the cork to allow escape of air or for suction to be applied. With effective intercostal drainage bubbling of air through the underwater seal is usually accompanied by re-expansion of the lung and blood may also be evacuated.

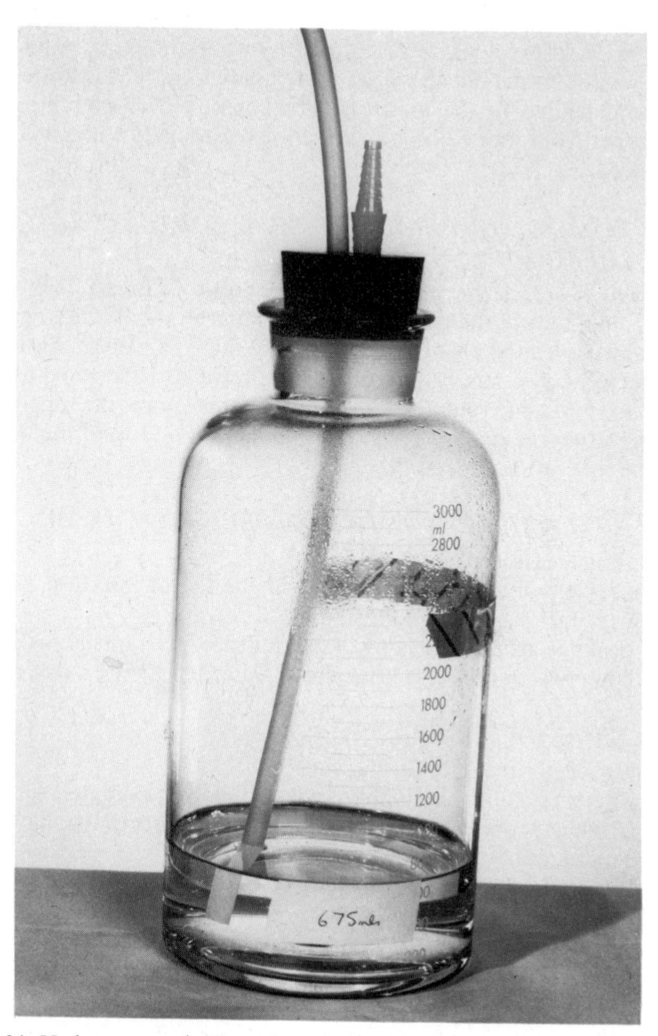

Fig. 24. Underwater seal. The nylon tubing which has superseded glass tubing readily distorts with high temperature sterilization, and may be so curved that its end may not reach the water level.

Complications of Chest Drainage

ACCIDENTAL WITHDRAWAL OF TUBE FROM THE CHEST

This may occur if either the securing suture breaks or loosens, or it may be withdrawn as a result of clumsy bedmaking. This has happened when patients have sat up for radiography whilst the tube has been pinned to the mattress. The consequences of tube withdrawal are from time to time quite serious, especially when this goes unnoticed.

SIPHONING OF UNDERWATER SEAL CONTENTS INTO THE CHEST

This will occur if the underwater seal bottle is raised to a level higher than that of the patient when the water in the bottle (together with any associated disinfectant) will pass into the pleura. Although this accident now rarely happens in the ward it may from time to time occur during the transport of patients from the operating theatre, when the underwater bottles are placed on top of the trolley and the tube is unclamped.

EXTERNAL AIR LEAK INTO THE PLEURAL CAVITY

a. Damaged tubing.
b. Leakage of air around the tube at the site of insertion.
c. Leakage at adaptor connections.
d. Leakage around the bung of the underwater drainage seal.
e. Underwater drainage tube above water level.

BLOCKAGE OF TUBES

This may occur at the following sites:
a. The chest tube may be blocked with clot or exudate.
b. The chest tube may be kinked or crushed beneath the mattress.
c. The tube may be inadvertently clamped.
d. Ineffective suction in the presence of a large air leak will have the same effect as clamping the tube.

If the air leak ceases and is associated with clinical and radiological expansion of the lung, it is well to leave the tube in place for a further 36 hours. It is useful to clamp the tube for 24 hours prior to removal, as this has the effect of removing the tube. A further radiograph just before tube removal ensures that further pneumothorax is not present, for if air has reaccumulated in the pleura the need for persistence of tube drainage is clear.

Air leak may continue for many days following chest injury. So long as the escape of air from the chest is as rapid as leakage from the lung and the lung remains expanded, there is little to cause concern, for sooner or later the damaged lung will seal and the leak cease. It is important to ensure that the tube is neither blocked nor displaced. A common cause of apparent air leak is that of air leaking into the chest through the stab wound and around the catheter. If this is suspected a further suture to tighten this wound is necessary.

Furious bubbling into the underwater seal indicates considerable air loss and simple drainage may be insufficient to prevent further pneumothorax. In this situation suction should be applied to the exit tube. The most useful type of sucker is a high volume, low pressure type, and if wall suction is used an appropriate reducing valve is necessary. It should be recognized that poor suction is more dangerous than free drainage, for whereas free drainage will always prevent a build up of tension pneumothorax inadequate suction may have the same effect as clamping the tube.

Indications for Thoracotomy

If despite efficient high volume suction the lung fails to re-expand, or the patient is clearly losing more air from his chest with each breath than his normal tidal volume, a large air leak from a lung tear or ruptured bronchus should be suspected. Subcutaneous emphysema may be prominent in the latter situation and suspicion of such damage should suggest that thoracotomy must not be long delayed.

CHRONIC PNEUMOTHORAX

Should the patient present some weeks after injury with a previously undiagnosed pneumothorax the subsequent pathology may preclude successful lung re-expansion. The pleural space commonly becomes infected and the consequent outpouring of protein induces the formation of a peel of fibrin, and later young fibrous tissue, on the surface of the lung. Certainly an initial attempt at tube drainage should be attempted, and this may be successful. However, in many cases the lung will fail to re-expand, and the persistence of tube drainage in this situation is not only futile but if prolonged will result in the formation of an empyema. The appropriate treatment of this condition is thoracotomy with decortication. The operator will be surprised to find considerable amounts of gelatinous protein and fibrin in the chest, together with large and unsuspected amounts of turbid fluid. The lung will be encased in an opaque membrane which prevents its re-expansion. Peeling the membrane from the lung is often tedious with the production of further considerable alveolar air leak and oozing from the lung surface, but following satisfactory decortication the lung will expand fully. The chest is closed with two pleural drains.

TRAUMATIC HAEMOTHORAX

Although commonly associated with pneumothorax, the problems presented by intrathoracic bleeding are worthy of further and separate consideration. A small amount of intrapleural bleeding usually accompanies chest injuries, although from time to time serious bleeding demands urgent attention. Such bleeding not only causes compression collapse of the lung but is associated with haemorrhagic shock. This may be complicated by the later development of clotted haemothorax, fibrothorax and empyema. Since each pleural cavity can, in an adult, contain up to 3 litres of blood, the patient may lose much of his blood volume internally.

Bleeding may originate from chest wall vessels (intercostals, internal mammaries and diaphragmatic), the lung or from the heart and great vessels. Although frequently occurring at the time of injury, the development of haemothorax may be delayed for many days, presumably by the displacement of rib fragments causing further damage.

Diagnosis

A small haemothorax may cause few if any symptoms and indeed pass unnoticed on physical examination. Radiologically there may be loss of the acute costophrenic angle together with a hazy appearance over the lower chest. Greater loss of blood shows itself more readily as the patient's general condition will suggest that blood loss has occurred and examination of the chest demonstrates the presence of fluid, which may be demonstrated radiologically. However, the radiological diagnosis of intrathoracic bleeding can be difficult, for even in the erect position as much as 500 ml of blood can be hidden behind the dome of the diaphragm. Changing the patient's position and performing the radiograph in the lateral decubitus position may demonstrate this blood loss.

Treatment

A small or moderate-sized haemothorax can be treated by chest aspiration using a wide bore chest needle and this may be repeated if necessary.

However, for many patients tube drainage is more effective and the patient is saved repeated attacks with the aspiration set. Certainly a combination of haemothorax and pneumothorax is best treated by intercostal catheter drainage. A large-bored siliconed catheter is inserted into the 6th intercostal space in the midaxillary line. The anterior aspect of the 2nd intercostal space is not recommended unless associated with pneumothorax for fear of introducing the trocar directly into the lung. Great care should be taken to avoid inserting the catheter too low in the chest or the liver, spleen or diaphragm may be damaged.

In most patients tube drainage will be sufficient. Despite the sometimes frightening initial blood loss when the tube is inserted, and this may amount to more than a litre, it usually soon ceases and with adequate blood replacement the patient's condition improves. Thoracotomy is rarely necessary in the early management of haemothorax, although from time to time the initial rapid drainage of blood may alarm the surgeon into performing a hasty, and perhaps unnecessary exploratory thoracotomy, for in most cases no active bleeding point will be found.

MASSIVE BLEEDING INTO THE CHEST

Surgical shock, dyspnoea and anoxia are prominent and associated with the physical signs of fluid in the chest and mediastinal displacement. Although the prompt insertion of a large-bored intercostal catheter will help to assess the amount of blood loss, it may be that the consequent lowering of intrapleural pressure will allow further serious bleeding from a large vessel. In this situation it is well to have facilities for thoracotomy readily available.

INDICATIONS FOR THORACOTOMY

The decision to explore the chest depends on such features as the amount of blood loss and its rate of reaccumulation, or the suspicion of damage to the heart and great vessels, lung or diaphragm. Although the decision to undertake thoracotomy is more common in the treatment of penetrating wounds, it does from time to time arise in closed injuries. Should the patient remain in a state of severe surgical shock which is unresponsive to blood transfusion exploration is indicated. In that situation thoracotomy or a combined thoraco-abdominal exploration may be required, for a ruptured spleen or a ruptured liver may be responsible.

CLOTTED HAEMOTHORAX

Occasionally a patient may present days or weeks following chest injury with a haemothorax resistant to simple drainage. Early organization of blood clot may have begun and a peel of fibrin will have developed over the lung, preventing its re-expansion. A peel

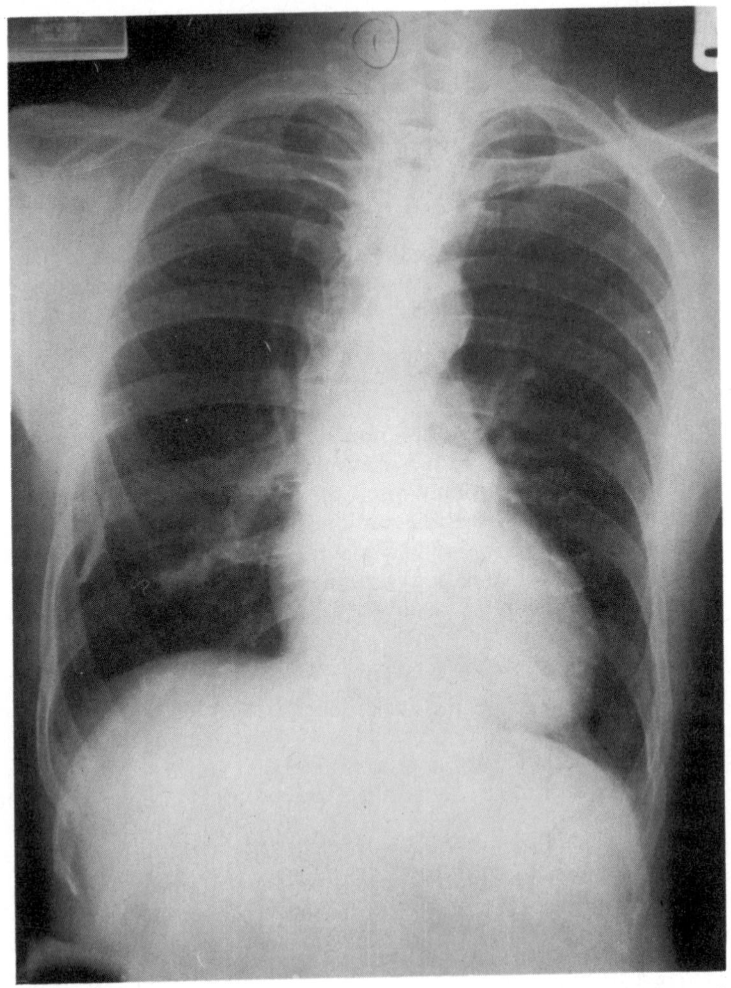

Fig. 25. This chest radiograph, which was taken shortly after the patient fell down a long flight of stairs, shows little amiss.

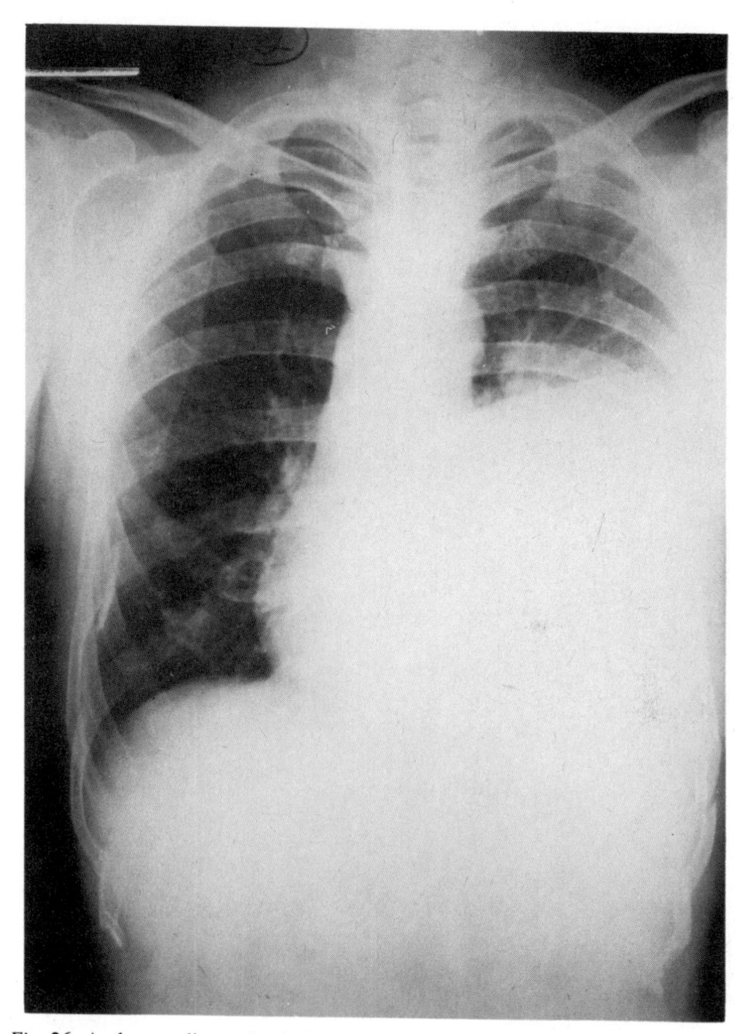

Fig. 26. A chest radiograph of the same patient shown in *Fig*. 25 2 weeks later demonstrates a lesion which was shown to be a large clotted haemothorax.

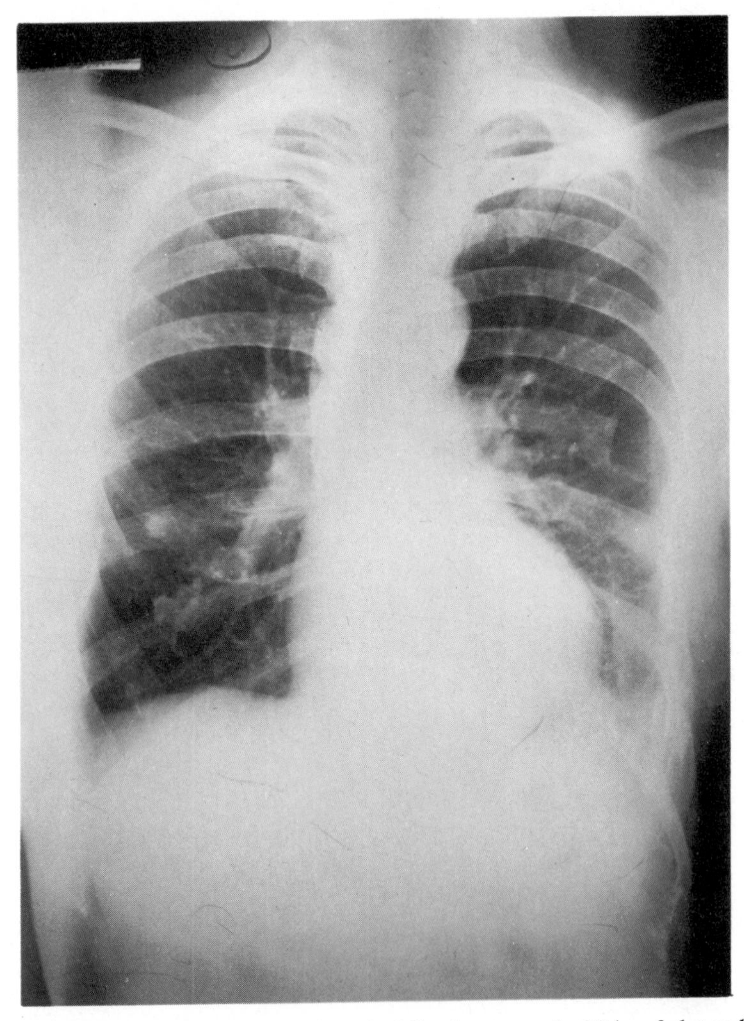

Fig. 27. Chest radiograph taken 2 weeks following removal of 2 kg of clot and decortication of the left lung. (*See Figs*. 25 and 26.)

also forms on the inner aspect of the chest wall and if untreated these layers organize and become thick fibrous tissue. The end-result may be a frozen and almost functionless hemithorax.

Treatment

Since drainage by means of a needle or an intercostal tube is impossible, it may be worth while to attempt to treat clotted haemothorax by the instillation of lytic enzymes such as streptokinase. These substances liquefy blood clot and later aspiration may be rewarded. Certainly persistent and repeated instillations of these substances for several weeks may be of value, and partial re-expansion of the lung and some degree of chest mobility may be restored. However, this is at the expense of pain, febrile systemic reactions to these enzymes, occasional empyema formation and usually incomplete drainage.

It is difficult to justify these weeks of unpleasant hospital treatment, accepting in the end a less than satisfactory result. It is better in such circumstances to undertake early thoracotomy. A short incision is adequate (15 cm), entering the chest through the 6th rib bed. The clot, which will have a placenta-like consistency, is removed, the fibrous coverings of the lung and chest wall peeled away, and the chest closed with drainage. The patient is ambulant following tube removal and may well be home within a week. Furthermore, normal respiratory function and full chest movements are to be anticipated, in contradistinction to those treated by aspiration and instillation of enzymes. (*See Figs.* 25–27.)

Chapter 8

Skeletal injuries and flail chest: fractured ribs and sternum

Fractures of the thoracic cage involving ribs or sternum may be of no serious consequence. More important is the intrathoracic damage which may have been sustained as part of the injury or the alteration in chest wall stability which may interfere with the mechanism of ventilation.

Treatment of pain may be difficult and it is important that the patient, especially if elderly or bronchitic, be encouraged to cough. Simple analgesics may help but if pain is severe infiltration with local anaesthetic solutions into the fracture site or the use of intercostal block or epidural anaesthesia may be invaluable (*see* Chapter 3). Although splinting of the chest wall with adhesive strapping may offer some relief this may encourage retention of secretions and is best avoided in elderly patients. It is important to repeat the chest radiograph 24 hours following injury to exclude pneumothorax or haemothorax. Fractures of the lower ribs, especially on the left side, may be associated with splenic rupture. Lower rib fractures may cause pain to be referred to the upper abdomen, the associated tenderness and rigidity giving rise to suspicion of splenic or hepatic injury which may be difficult to exclude. In this situation diagnostic peritoneal tap may be of assistance. Fracture of the 1st rib is rare and usually associated with fracture of the clavicle and adjacent ribs. This injury may be caused by severe downwards trauma against the clavicle and upper chest and is particularly dangerous as it may be associated with damage to the great vessels in that region.

Multiple fractures are commonly associated with great pain and marked spasm of the chest wall. Coughing is avoided and breathing

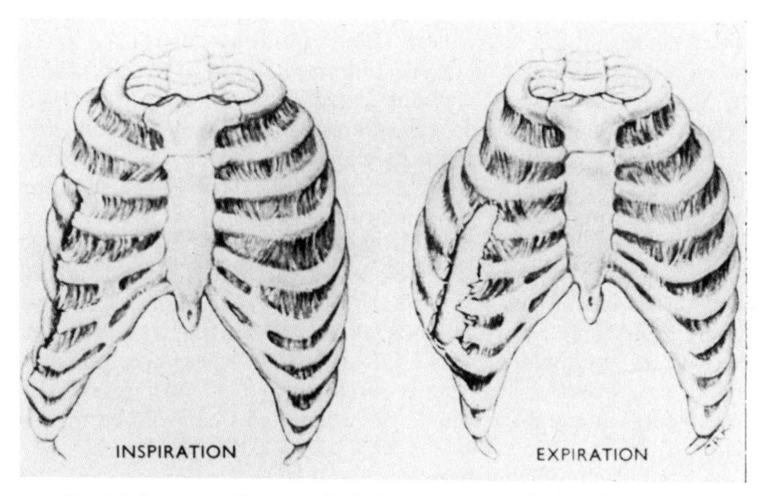

Fig. 28. Flail chest. The paradoxical movement of the flail segment is demonstrated.

may be grunting in type. The stage is set for atelectasis, and associated lung damage will aggravate the problem. Treatment is directed toward the painless expulsion of secretions.

FLAIL CHEST (*Fig*. 28)

When two or more ribs are fractured in two places or are fractured posteriorly with sternochondral dislocation anteriorly, the flail panel renders the chest wall unstable, interfering with the mechanics of ventilation; the larger the flail panel the greater is such interference. The mobile segment moves abnormally, being sucked in on inspiration and thrust out with expiration: that is, the segment moves paradoxically. Such paradoxical movement interferes with the patient's ability to create a negative intrapleural pressure and consequently the tidal volume falls considerably. The patient needs to breathe more rapidly to achieve oxygenation but anoxia and carbon dioxide retention supervene. This is followed by exhaustion and, if unrelieved, death commonly follows.

It was formerly believed that the respiratory difficulty associated with 'stove-in' chest was caused by a pendulum movement of air from one lung to the other, so called *Pendelluft*. The early thoracic surgeons noted that after the operation of thoracoplasty the decostalized portion of the chest wall moved in a direction opposite to that of the remainder of the thorax, being sucked in on inspiration and pushed out on expiration. The respiratory distress in these patients was attributed to the pendulum-like motion of gases from one lung to the other. It was postulated that with each inspiration oxygen and carbon dioxide passed from the lung on the flail side into the normal lung and during expiration the process was considered to be reversed. This concept of *Pendelluft* was accepted for many years and taught to generations of students, but there is good clinical and experimental evidence to suggest that the concept of *Pendelluft* be abandoned (Maloney et al., 1961). A more likely explanation is that both pleural cavities work as a single bellows system rather than as two independent chambers. Clearly damage to the bellows interferes with its ability to induce a negative pressure and if the 'stove-in' segment is large enough its own to-and-fro movement will equal in volume the attempted tidal volume of the bellows.

In many such afflicted patients, paradoxical movement may not appear for some time, for a combination of muscle spasm and impaction of the broken rib ends may splint the segment. However, as spasm wears off and the fragments loosen paradox appears. Effective coughing becomes impossible for it is difficult to build up the required 'head of pressure' to expel secretions forcibly and atelectasis may follow. If the flail segment is anterior or lateral it is usually of serious consequence for in these situations it is unsupported. On the other hand, a posterior flail segment is often well supported by the thick overlying muscles and the scapula. It is therefore rarely accompanied by important respiratory complications (*Fig*. 29).

Flail chest is usually associated with other major trauma and associated head or skeletal injuries are frequent. Furthermore, haemothorax, pneumothorax and lung contusions may complicate an already serious injury.

Treatment of Flail Chest

The principles of treatment are:

1. Restitution of adequate ventilation.
2. Maintenance of clear airway.
3. Stabilization of the flail segment.

At the roadside the violently breathing anoxic patient is best helped by rolling him on to the affected side, perhaps with a rolled coat or sandbag under the flail segment. This has the effect of splinting the segment and to some extent controls the paradoxical movement, enabling the patient to take deeper, more efficient breaths

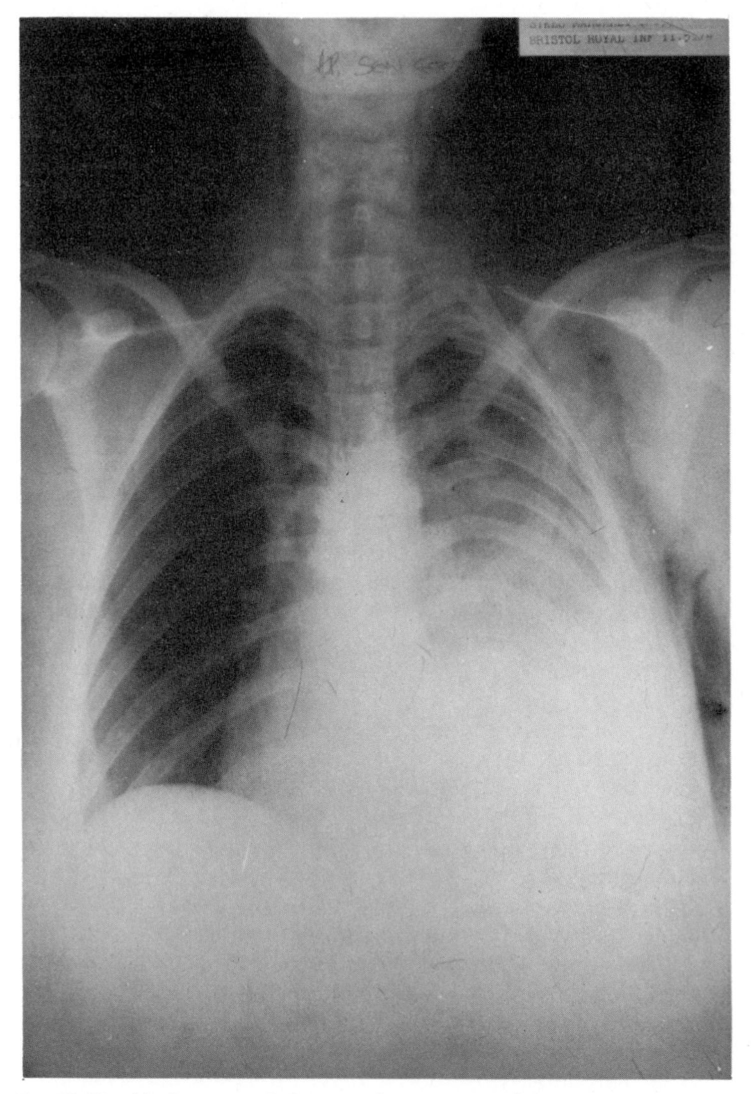

Fig. 29. Double fractures of the posterior segments of the upper 5 ribs on the left side. Despite this mobile fragment a flail situation did not result owing to the supportive action of the chest wall muscles in this area.

with consequent improvement in oxygenation. In the young and fit minor degrees of flail chest have been treated by compression of the segment by a pad held in place by elastic strapping, but this has the disadvantage of impairing ventilation and coughing, predisposing to atelectasis. In an emergency towel clips passed through the skin to encircle one or more ribs within the flail segment and fixed to a traction device may stabilize the segment. Although this measure has been improved to include elaborate arrangements using pulleys attached to a Balkan frame and supported by weights, these methods are cumbersome and largely obsolete. Such a system may appear attractive in a photograph but has great disadvantages in practice and furthermore tissue necrosis and infection commonly occur. In deciding on the need for stabilization two questions should be asked:

1. Can the patient breathe adequately?
2. Can he cough effectively?

Adequacy of ventilation may be difficult to assess for not only the rate and depth of ventilation but, more important, the work of ventilation must be considered. Measurements of tidal volume and minute volume may be extremely helpful but may be misleading in the absence of close observation of the patient.

Serial blood gas analysis is of great value indicating improvement or deterioration and giving valuable supportive evidence of the state of the patient. With experience it is not difficult to recognize those patients who need ventilatory assistance, but the following observations taken together or separately may be regarded as confirmatory evidence:

1. Low tidal volume and decreasing tidal volume.
2. Low vital capacity.
3. Excessive respiratory effort.
4. Low and falling $P\text{ao}_2$.
5. High and rising $P\text{co}_2$.
6. Low venous $P\text{o}_2$.

In 1956 Avery et al. made a most important contribution to the treatment of the crushed chest. Like others, they had observed that many patients could be maintained over prolonged periods by means of intermittent positive pressure ventilation via a tracheostomy, particularly in the treatment of tetanus and poliomyelitis. They were encouraged by the observation that a number of their own patients with severe chest injuries, who were rapidly failing with the methods of treatment at that time, quickly stabilized and eventually recovered with the use of continuous mechanical ventilation, using a piston-type intermittent positive pressure respirator which had been developed by Mörch in 1940, in Copenhagen. They considered that this novel method was safe and allowed survival of patients with a seemingly hopeless prognosis. They noted that other benefits included correction of paradoxical movement of the chest wall, relief of hypoxia and hypercarbia, together with a reduction of the need for powerful sedation. They concluded that continuous mechanical ventilation should find a much wider range of application where there is loss of integrity of the chest wall, severe infection, neurological disease and muscle disease, head injuries and drug overdosage. They noted that these patients died not of these primary pathological conditions but of the complications of decreased pulmonary ventilation. Their case report and observations were a landmark in the treatment of chest injuries and clearly placed them ahead of their time.

The views of Barrett (1960) are of interest for at that time this injury was poorly understood and its treatment by artificial ventilation was just gaining ground. He pointed out that patients with multiple injuries which included a 'stove-in' chest often died without obvious cause: 'Haemorrhage has been stemmed, transfusions have been given and ample morphine has relieved the pain. The sedated patient lies quietly in bed and his shallow paradoxical respiratory movements escape critical notice but death steps in suddenly, peacefully, naturally and unnecessarily.' Barrett was among the first to advocate forcefully the advantages and merits of intermittent positive pressure ventilation in this condition.

When the chest wall is badly crushed, particularly bilaterally, adequate stabilization may be provided by intermittent positive pressure ventilation, by internal fixation of ribs, or by a combination of these methods, and the advantages and disadvantages of these methods will be discussed on page 73. The concept of providing intermittent positive pressure to patients with ventilatory insufficiency is not new. Positive pressure and negative pressure cabinets were developed by Brauer and Sauerbruch many years ago. More recently a large variety of useful and effective positive pressure ventilators have been developed, the stimulus for their production being the severe epidemic of poliomyelitis in the middle 1940s. Since the publication of the classic paper of Avery et al. (1956) numerous reports of large series of patients with crushed chests treated in this way have emerged, and the success of intermittent positive pressure ventilation in the treatment of these patients has gained wide acceptance.

However, there is little doubt that whereas artificial ventilation for prolonged periods is well tolerated by young patients, the mortality and morbidity when used in the elderly and bronchitic are extremely high. The very real hazards of prolonged intermittent positive pressure ventilation, either by endotracheal tube or via a tracheostomy, in the elderly cannot be overlooked for it is in this group that the mortality may be as high as 50 per cent in patients over the age of 60. It is these considerations which prompt the protagonists of surgical fixation away from prolonged artificial ventilation in elderly patients, for in these patients a flail segment may from time to time be adequately fixed by nailing or wiring, thus eliminating the need for or reducing the period of intermittent positive pressure ventilation.

Bickford and his colleagues (1974), reviewing their series of 88 patients with chest injuries treated over a 5-year period, reported an overall death rate of 12·5 per cent. Of their whole series 25 per cent required tracheostomy and 19 needed to be ventilated mechanically. Of the latter 7 died and the mortality over the age of 50 was very much greater (75 per cent) than in younger patients (9 per cent). Mortality in their patients was related to the severity of the injury, especially if there was an initial contusion of the lungs. Infection with Gram-negative organisms following intermittent positive pressure ventilation was frequently fatal in their older patients. They concluded that intermittent positive pressure ventilation should be avoided whenever possible, perhaps by the wider use of surgical stabilization of the chest. They pointed out, however, that it is very difficult to suggest an adequate alternative for many of these severely injured patients. This last remark takes us to the very root of this debate, for no matter how sincerely we may believe artificial ventilation to be deleterious it is clearly not possible to watch these patients die for lack of it.

It has been suggested that should thoracotomy be inevitable (such as for the repair of ruptured diaphragm) the opportunity should be taken to nail or wire the fractured ribs. Certainly in this situation the temptation to do so is great but it is unfortunate that such opportunities are rare and form a very small proportion of these injuries. The crushed chest is rarely a simple problem of either flail chest or haemothorax or pneumothorax or pulmonary contusions. Frequently two or more of these conditions coexist and furthermore may be bilateral. The addition of a head injury or a major fracture is by no means uncommon. It is very unusual for a flail chest to be the sole injury in an otherwise unblemished patient. For the majority, therefore, internal operative fixation of fractured ribs is an unrealistic approach, for despite the mechanical stability sometimes achieved by these methods it is inevitable that concomitant chest injuries and the effect of a long operation make a period of intermittent positive pressure ventilation unavoidable. Surgical fixation of the flail chest should not be considered an alternative to intermittent positive pressure ventilation solely for the reason that the admitting hospital lacks facilities for prolonged artificial ventilation. In such circumstances the patient should be intubated, ventilated and resuscitated overnight and then removed at the earliest safe time to the nearest hospital with a special care unit. In 1961 Windsor and Dwyer reported the success of moving such injured patients by air in Australia and observed this to be an entirely reasonable and practical approach.

Hospitals lacking a special care unit and a group of anaesthetists and nurses prepared to manage such a patient by prolonged artificial ventilation are unlikely to carry a surgeon capable of either assessing the injury or of undertaking adequate fixative surgery. Although photographs, and particularly diagrams, may convey the impression that these operations are simple and effective procedures, the wide and difficult exposure necessary forms no part of the experience of those untrained in thoracic surgery. In the hands of thoracic surgeons the results of these procedures frequently fall short of ideal, for the ribs are often so comminuted that fixation of the mobile fragments is difficult. Despite such surgical fixation, intermittent positive pressure ventilation may be necessary for a short time.

Severe compression or deceleration injuries applied to the front of the chest may fracture all or most of the ribs, costal cartilages or sternocostal junctions unilaterally or bilaterally. When bilateral, the chest becomes unstable on account of this floating sternal segment. Although many patients respond to simple measures or to artificial ventilation this is an ideal situation for the use of internal fixation which is both simple and effective. A stainless-steel strip about 20 cm long and 1 cm wide is so placed that its centre is behind the sternum and its ends anterior to the chest wall. Stability is excellent and derives from a well-tried method of achieving stability after the surgical correction of funnel chest. The steel strip may be left in place indefinitely or removed by way of a small incision several months later.

Internal Fixation of Flail Chest

Although intermittent positive pressure ventilation is a satisfactory method of treating flail chest in younger patients, the complications of this treatment in elderly people and the consequent morbidity and high mortality have persuaded many surgeons to adopt an aggressive policy of internal stabilization of the individual fractures of the ribs, costal cartilages and the sternum using various wires, nails or splints. There are now a number of surgeons who electively use this method in the management of isolated flail chest and whose long term results have certainly been as good as or better than the management of elderly patients using intermittent positive pressure ventilation alone. In 1977 Moore reported his results in 68 patients who were treated in the 19-year period from 1958 to 1977. He reported an overall mortality of 14 patients (20·5 per cent). However, the mortality in 10 patients over 70 years of age was 5 (50 per cent) and in most of these death was due to causes other than the chest injury. In his series a very high proportion of flail chests in patients over the age of 70 and even younger were due to falls, which on closer investigation were shown to be due to aortic stenosis, cerebral atherosclerosis and other degenerative processes. At the other extremes of age, that is in patients under the age of 20 years, the chest wall was usually so elastic that blunt injuries to the chest produced severe visceral damage with only mild or moderate degrees of flail chest injuries. Several of these young patients died of lacerated lungs due to closed injuries but with only moderate degrees of flail chest.

Moore was therefore tempted to make a valid comparison of different modes of management of flail chest and selected patients aged between 25 and 65 years of age. He avoided tracheostomy in all but 12 of his 68 patients. In 4 it was used to aspirate the secretions only in unconscious or feeble patients, and in 8 others positive pressure ventilation was used in addition to internal fixation but for relatively short periods. Two further patients required positive pressure ventilation for longer than 48 hours postoperatively, one for 5 and one for 10 days. Scrutiny of those 14 patients who required intermittent positive pressure ventilation revealed that 6 were in coma and 1 confused and 3 others had the tracheostomy performed before admission. Of the remaining 4, 1 was aged 77 years, 2 had severe emphysema, and the last a fractured mandible and a compound comminuted fracture of the femur, which may have caused pulmonary fat embolism. Six of these 14 patients died and there was no complication of tracheostomy in his series. Moore concluded from the study of his limited series that positive pressure ventilation for more than 48 hours by endotracheal tube can be avoided in the worst cases of flail chest, other than in the elderly and those with brain damage and those with substantial pre-existing lung disease or other associated serious injuries.

In the follow-up of his 54 survivors the clinical state concerning respiratory function and deformity was satisfactory in the majority, and he expressed the hope that more thoracic surgeons would undertake this more aggressive but in his view safer method of internal fixation rather than resort to intermittent positive pressure ventilation in all patients.

TECHNIQUE OF INTERNAL FIXATION

The surgical approach is through an anterolateral or postero-lateral thoracotomy reflecting the shoulder girdle and scapula away from the chest wall, exposing the anterior and posterior aspects of the fractured ribs. These are then fixed using either Kirschner wires or Rush nails, and the pleura is opened to remove blood clots and other fluid and in order to insert chest tubes.

CONCLUSIONS

There is little doubt that most patients with flail chest are best treated by artificial ventilation, internal fixation being reserved for elderly patients in whom the anatomy of the injury is suitable for such repair. With artificial ventilation it should be anticipated that a period of at least 10 days of treatment will be required. Although an endotracheal tube may prove adequate, tracheostomy may be necessary should treatment be prolonged or there be a severe concomitant head injury or facio-maxillary injury.

With improvements in equipment, respiratory care techniques and nursing skills, satisfactory survival rates have been achieved with the increased use of artificial ventilation in chest injuries severe enough to cause respiratory failure. While it is true that artificial ventilation should not be employed when simpler means will suffice, it is equally true that the judicious and early use of artificial ventilation in these patients will lead to improved survival rates.

FRACTURES OF THE STERNUM

These are uncommon following either direct violence to the chest or a hyperflexion injury associated with crush fractures of the vertebral bodies. Since the majority of sternal fractures are associated with the steering wheel type of injury, the mortality rate associated may be high, due to the severity of associated injuries. A blow severe enough to fracture the sternum is frequently associated with rupture of the aorta, major air passages or diaphragm, and an associated flail chest or myocardial injury is common, as are associated head injuries.

Most sternal fractures occur in the body at or near its junction with the manubrium and the synchondrosis between these may be separated (*Fig.* 30). They are usually transverse and if displaced the upper segment lies behind the lower fragment. The posterior

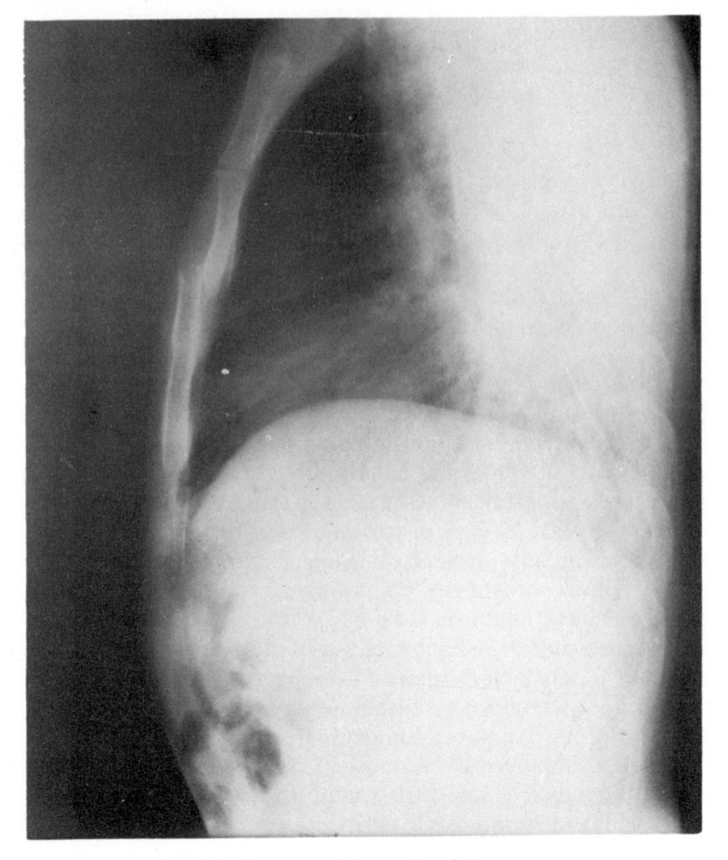

Fig. 30. Fracture of the body of the sternum.

periosteum is usually intact accounting for the stability and good union associated with this injury. Pain and tenderness are prominent and if mobile the pain may be severe. Impacted fractures may pass unnoticed in the presence of other injuries. Radiologically they may be missed unless a lateral film is taken which is diagnostic.

Treatment

Undisplaced sternal fractures are best treated by analgesics and the local injection of anaesthetic is convenient and rewarding. Although bed-rest for 2–3 weeks lying flat is advocated by some, there is no doubt that early ambulation is desirable and the patient should be out of bed as soon as other injuries permit. A displaced fracture may sometimes be reduced by hyperextension of the spine with the arms extended over the head, at the same time pressing backwards on the lower fragment. General anaesthesia is required for this manœuvre. Pain from an excessively mobile fracture may justify the reduction and perhaps fixation of some of these fractures, but it is neither necessary nor desirable to interfere with these fractures for they will usually heal satisfactorily with neither deformity nor residual symptoms.

If operative reduction and fixation are required, wiring the fragments together is readily achieved but it is particularly in these mobile fragments that further postoperative displacement may readily occur.

TRAUMATIC LUNG HERNIA

Lung hernias are rare and occur in the cervical position, penetrating Sibson's fascia in about one-third of the cases. The remainder appear through the chest wall. Although some lung hernias are congenital trauma seems to be the commonest cause. The indications for surgery depend on the severity of symptoms. Should a large cervical hernia need reduction and repair it is clearly more practical to approach this via the transthoracic route, for an adequate exposure of Sibson's fascia from above is extremely difficult. At thoracotomy the edges of the defect are clearly seen and it is best closed off using a sheet of woven Dacron which is sutured carefully to the edges of the defect (Lightwood and Cleland, 1974).

Chapter 9

Lung injuries

Although lung damage is associated with penetrating injuries, it is common for a significant degree of such damage to accompany closed trauma. Pathological conditions include lacerations, contusions and so-called 'traumatic wet lung'. Although pulmonary embolism and fat embolism may complicate chest injuries and indeed cause death, a discussion of these conditions is not included here.

LACERATION OF THE LUNG

Since the pulmonary artery pressure is less than one-third of the systemic arterial pressure, bleeding from lacerations is less likely to be significant than elsewhere. The damaged portion of lung rapidly becomes oedematous and solid, resembling liver in appearance and consistency, helping to seal off torn vessels. The air leak, however, stops less readily. Lacerations vary in severity from near avulsion of a lung or lobe to short pleural splits. The effect of such lacerations is related to the degree of air leak and haemorrhage produced. The symptoms, signs and investigation of associated pneumothorax and haemothorax have been reviewed, and in most patients with a laceration of the lung, intercostal catheter drainage will have been instituted. The majority of smaller lacerations respond to this management, the air leak closing and bleeding ceasing. There is healing in most cases without significant loss of lung function.

Should bleeding via the intercostal tube be severe or should massive haemothorax present together with shock, thoracotomy may be necessary and from time to time serious and continued air leak will require exploration. In both of these cases a lacerated lung may be responsible for the lesion.

At thoracotomy it is important to preserve lung tissue, sacrificing only that which is clearly avascular or almost detached. The surgeon should not feel impelled to remove a badly bruised lobe, for such damage is capable of complete resolution with little loss of function. Air leaks should be oversewn and small leaking air passages tied off. Bleeding vessels require ligature or coagulation. The torn lung is then reconstructed by lightly suturing or stapling the torn pleural edges together. From time to time severe bleeding is seen to originate from major pulmonary vessels and when associated with a large air leak, problems of exposure and control become complicated. This situation is more readily remedied by controlling the lung hilum with a shod gastro-intestinal clamp or a light vascular clamp. It is necessary to include the pulmonary artery and veins together with the bronchus in this clamping, after which bleeding and air leak are dramatically reduced and careful exposure of torn vessels is then straightforward. These should, if at all possible, be repaired with fine vascular sutures and it is surprising how readily an almost completely avulsed large vessel can be reconstituted.

Despite attempts to conserve lung tissue it may rarely be necessary to undertake emergency lobectomy or pneumonectomy.

CASE REPORT

An 8-year-old boy was struck by a car in the left chest with consequent multiple rib fractures. He was admitted to hospital with severe haemoptysis complicated by aspiration of blood into the good lung, and within a short time his condition deteriorated with severe cyanosis and circulatory failure. He was anaesthetized and intubated, and this was followed by further blood loss which was aspirated from the endotracheal tube at a constant and alarming rate. Left thoracotomy was undertaken 1 hour after injury. The left lower lobe was solid and red with obvious disruption of its substance. The interlobar fissure was exposed and compression of the pulmonary artery within the fissure was rewarded by cessation of bleeding from the endotracheal tube. It appeared that the pulmonary vessels were torn and bleeding within the lung parenchyma. Left lower lobectomy was undertaken with improvement in the child's general condition. The post-operative course was stormy for the residual left lung and the right lung contained inhaled blood, but following several days of artificial ventilation radiological resolution took place which was followed by recovery.

LUNG CONTUSION (*Fig.* 31)

This is the description given to the radiological appearance of small or larger fluffy patches which may become confluent and bilateral. It says little of the pathological processes but it is nevertheless associated with serious consequences when widespread. Contusion follows direct trauma to the lung or may affect the opposite lung, a

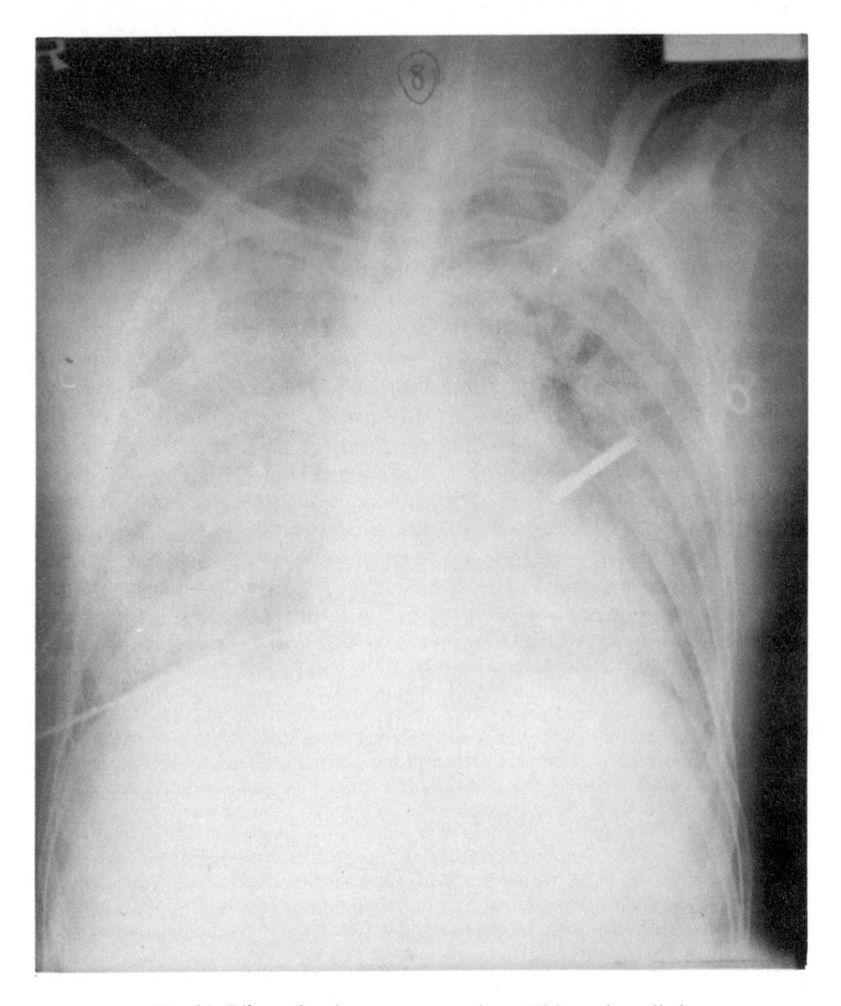

Fig. 31. Bilateral pulmonary contusions. This patient died.

so-called *contre-coup* effect. The massive lung contusions of blast injuries which accompany both shotgun and high velocity, small missile wounds are frequently severe enough to cause fatal anoxia.

Pathology

A mixture of oedema, interstitial and alveolar haemorrhage, together with atelectasis and thrombosis, is responsible for the radiological appearance, and macroscopically the affected portions of lung are purple and solid. Such damage is radiologically and probably also functionally completely recoverable, although the presence of severe and extensive contusions may so interfere with respiratory function that death occurs.

Treatment

Any chest injury will be aggravated by lung contusion. In addition to loss of respiratory function, oedema and contusion intefere with pulmonary compliance, increasing the work of respiration. Initially this may be adequately compensated but anoxia with carbon dioxide retention may follow. Expulsion of secretions is difficult, compounding an already precarious situation and exhaustion may follow. If it seems clear that anoxia and CO_2 retention are developing and that ventilation is inadequate, intermittent positive pressure ventilation via an endotracheal tube is necessary (*Fig.* 32). This ensures that the work of ventilation is removed from the patient, collapsed lung re-expanded and that secretions can be aspirated. This treatment is designed to make the maximum use of undamaged lung until resolution of the contused lung occurs. Such treatment may be necessary for some days. However, the contusions may enlarge and become more confluent radiologically and be associated with decreased pulmonary compliance. Despite adequate ventilation, arterial oxygen tension may fall to seemingly impossible low levels with concomitant rise in carbon dioxide tension, and in due course tissue anoxia is followed by metabolic acidosis and death.

It is rarely possible to succeed in such a critical situation and other forms of treatment are attempted from time to time. One such treatment is that of temporary artificial oxygenation.

ARTIFICIAL OXYGENATION

This is undertaken using a low volume high efficiency oxygenator. Since it is to be used in an extracorporeal blood circuit for several days it is recommended that the least haemotraumatic oxygenator available is used. The membrane oxygenator familiar to cardiac surgeons has proved ideal in these circumstances.

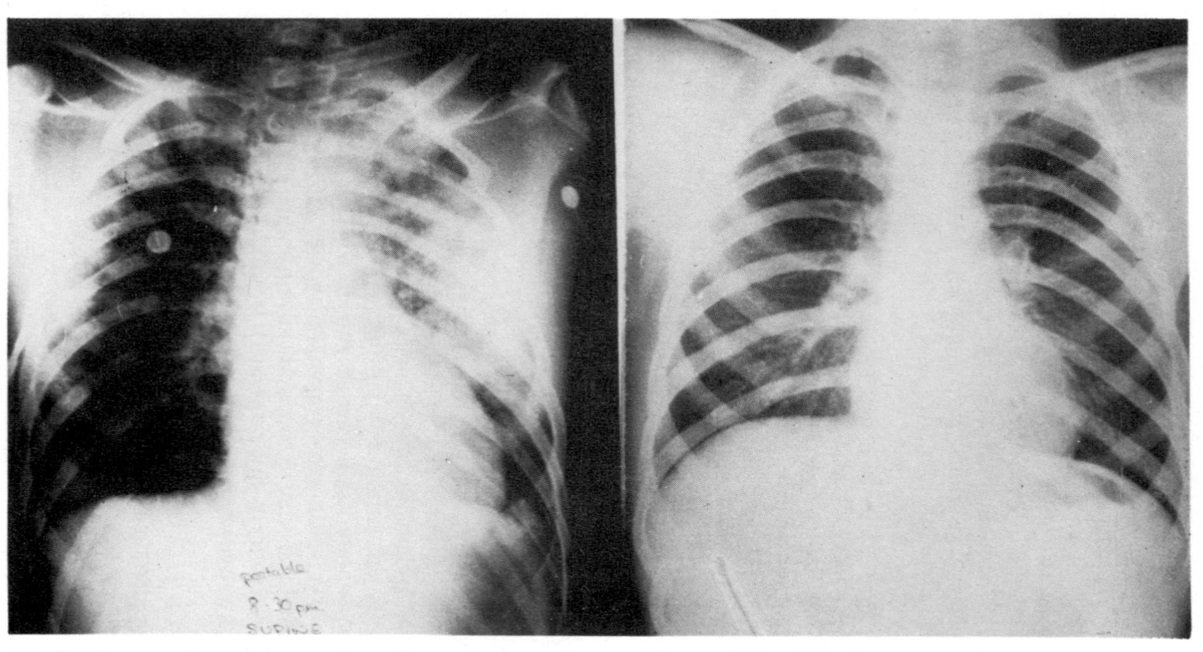

Fig. 32. Severe pulmonary contusions. The patient was dangerously anoxic but following 5 days of intermittent positive pressure ventilation his clinical condition improved dramatically and his chest radiograph demonstrated considerable clearing.

Perfusion may be performed via the femoral vessels, removing blood from the inferior vena cava with return to the femoral artery, although more recently the oxygenated blood has been returned to the internal jugular vein rather than the arterial system, thus avoiding the dangers of arterial air embolism and prolonged ischaemic changes in the limb. Low flow rates have been found to produce a significant elevation of $Pa\text{O}_2$ with consequent improvement of tissue perfusion. It is clearly unnecessary to aim at a high oxygen tension in the blood, for these patients come to treatment with a $Pa\text{O}_2$ of around 30 mmHg and elevation of this level to 65 mmHg is clinically clearly beneficial. It is important to manage with as low a flow rate as is possible, for blood and tissue damage are directly related to both flow rate and the duration of by-pass, and it may be necessary to maintain this perfusion for several days. In practice it has been found that a flow rate of about 2 litres per minute is satisfactory, elevating the $Pa\text{O}_2$ to safe levels and at the same time causing minimal blood damage.

One group of workers believe that should the ventilator inflation pressure be in excess of 40 cm of water and the $Pa\text{O}_2$ tension fall below 35 mmHg, death is inevitable, and that long term partial perfusion is indicated (Clarke, 1975).

Prolonged perfusion for periods of up to 5 days has been used in the treatment of pulmonary contusion, massive pulmonary fat embolism, respiratory burns, traumatic shock lung and post-operatively following cardiac surgery, and although the results are as yet disappointing, the few notable successes so far recorded should give encouragement to surgical teams treating these conditions (Hill, De Leval et al., 1972; Hill, O'Brien et al., 1972).

TRAUMATIC WET LUNG

This comprehensive term was introduced during World War II by military surgeons who noted that chest injuries were often accompanied by retention and accumulation of oedema, blood and secretions in the lung. Respiratory difficulty and cyanosis were noted and on listening to the chest diffuse râles were heard. The mechanism of this condition was unclear at that time, but was considered in some way to be associated with chest wall and broncho-pulmonary neurogenic reflexes. This latter explanation derives from the results of animal experiments in which blunt chest trauma is associated with bronchospasm, oedema and anoxia. It was considered that pulmonary capillary permeability may in some way be altered increasing the liability to oedema. Such chest injury was greatly feared, for it was frequently fatal. However, at that time little was known of assisted ventilation and knowledge of the treatment of chest injuries was restricted to a few specialists. Other terms such as 'traumatic stiff lung' and 'shock lung' probably described a similar process.

It seems possible that this condition is a combination of pulmonary contusion, atelectasis and oedema, perhaps complicated by aspiration of gastric contents. Today these conditions are the well-understood results of severe chest injuries and it may be that the term 'traumatic wet lung' is too generalized. Poorly understood damage to the pulmonary surfactant systems can undoubtedly produce in injured people a condition similar to that in respiratory distress of the newborn. Severe hypoxaemia due to diffusion problems may be improved by intermittent positive pressure ventilation, or rarely by recourse to artificial oxygenation.

Chapter 10

Tracheobronchial injuries

Although closed injuries of the main air passages are rare, most traumatic surgeons will eventually see such a case. This injury usually accompanies high speed car accidents and is particularly associated with the head-on collision in which the driver is decelerated by the steering wheel. It is likely that in addition to the shearing effect of violent deceleration such tears may be caused by high pressure internal 'explosions' of the large air passages. Crushing injuries and sudden burial by earth falls may be associated with this injury. Lloyd et al. (1958) subjected a series of anaesthetized dogs to closed trauma by dropping a 50-lb sandbag from a distance of 10 feet on to the chest. They found that in those animals with an open airway bronchial tears occurred in 15 per cent whereas in those animals in which the airway was closed by clamping the endotracheal tube the rate of bronchial rupture rose to 70 per cent. Whether or not disruptive forces damage the bronchus by forcibly separating the lungs is speculative but the role of the closed glottis in these accidents seems clear.

Rupture of the bronchus was reported in 1848 following a road traffic accident in which a pedestrian was run over by a cart (Webb, 1848) and again in 1863 involving a drunken horseman who was thrown (Biermer, 1863). This latter patient survived 22 days with massive subcutaneous emphysema and at autopsy there was complete transection of the left main bronchus with 3-cm separation of the ends. Kinsella and Johnsrud (1947) reported 38 cases from the literature and added 2 of their own. An analysis of this group showed that 4 patients died immediately and a further 5 within 1 hour of injury. These died because of associated injuries such as ruptured aorta, severed spinal cord or trachea or other injuries incompatible with life. Others who survived the immediate crisis died later of tension pneumothorax or haemorrhage.

Krinitzki reported the first known recovery from this injury in 1928, and in 1949 Griffith reported the first resection and re-anastomosis of a post-traumatic bronchial stricture. Scannell, in 1951, reported the successful repair of a ruptured bronchus within 3 hours of injury, since which time the clinical picture has been frequently described. Most reports of these injuries note the significant lack of damage to pulmonary vessels, supporting the view that bronchial rupture may be caused by high intrabronchial pressures rather than more direct trauma.

Penetrating injury of the bronchus is rare but Sanger (1945) reported 2 patients wounded at Anzio in 1944 who had suffered rupture of the left main bronchus by shell fragments. In both of these patients repair was possible, one by direct suture and in the other using sutures reinforced by a free muscle graft.

Diagnosis

Rupture of the bronchus presents either early as a surgical emergency or later with a fully developed bronchial stricture. Diagnosis may be delayed for this is a rare injury and pulmonary lacerations can produce a similar clinical picture. Furthermore, associated major injuries are common and divert attention elsewhere.

Complete rupture of the bronchus presents in a dramatic fashion but incomplete tears may remain silent until the development of bronchostenosis. Bishop et al. (1960), in a review of 80 patients with bronchial injury, noted pneumothorax in 59 per cent, tension pneumothorax in 16 per cent, severe dyspnoea in 48 per cent, subcutaneous emphysema in 39 per cent and rapidly progressive subcutaneous emphysema in 4 per cent. Only 40 per cent of their patients had broken ribs.

Traumatic pneumothorax is more usually caused by lung laceration and responds to catheter drainage, but a continued leak of large volumes of air should arouse the suspicion of bronchial tear. Whereas in the majority of patients with subcutaneous emphysema no serious pulmonary injury is present, the very rapid accumulation of subcutaneous emphysema might suggest rupture of the bronchus.

Diagnosis may be confirmed at bronchoscopy, for the majority of such tears, both complete and incomplete, can readily be seen. Bronchoscopy will determine the side of rupture and thus the elective side for exploratory thoracotomy. Bishop found that in

78 per cent of his cases diagnosis and repair were delayed for more than 1 week after injury but despite this repair was usually possible. Long delay is invariably followed by stricture, the patient presenting with stridor and pulmonary collapse and infection distal to the stricture. The diagnosis of stricture is made at bronchoscopy and by bronchography.

Treatment

Operative repair will vary in complexity from that of a few sutures in order to close a small bronchial tear to that of major mobilization of the trachea and both bronchi in order to repair a large laceration or rejoin an avulsed bronchus. Ingenious intubation and anaesthetic techniques need to be tailored at the time of operation to the needs of the injury. Having regard to other accompanying injuries, the sooner bronchial repair is undertaken the better. When early repair is not practical, delay of several weeks will permit resolution of acute oedema and allow more opportunity for healing without stricture formation.

Although incomplete tears may heal without stricture formation, strictures may be complicated by distal lung suppuration, abscess formation and lung destruction. The treatment of bronchial stricture by repeated bronchoscopic dilatation is not recommended, for this is inevitably followed by further and more resistant stricture formation. Resection of all post-traumatic strictures should be considered, for the distal lung remains permanently at risk of suppuration. Several authors have reported good functional results following resection of such strictures as long as 11 years following the causative accident (Mahaffey et al., 1956).

Whether repairing a bronchial tear at an early stage or resecting a stricture at a late one, it is important to remove dead cartilage and to trim the bronchus until free bleeding occurs. Suturing with interrupted stainless-steel wire or Prolene (polypropylene) is recommended. An appreciable postoperative air leak is common and adequate intercostal catheter drainage is necessary.

CASE REPORTS

1. A 10-year-old boy was buried face downwards by a fall of earth. He was resuscitated and admitted to a local hospital. Chest X-ray taken within 2 hours of injury demonstrated a left tension pneumothorax (*Fig.* 33). After the introduction of an intercostal catheter into the left pleural cavity a large quantity of air escaped and then the patient's condition improved. By the following day, although the patient appeared well, there was marked subcutaneous emphysema

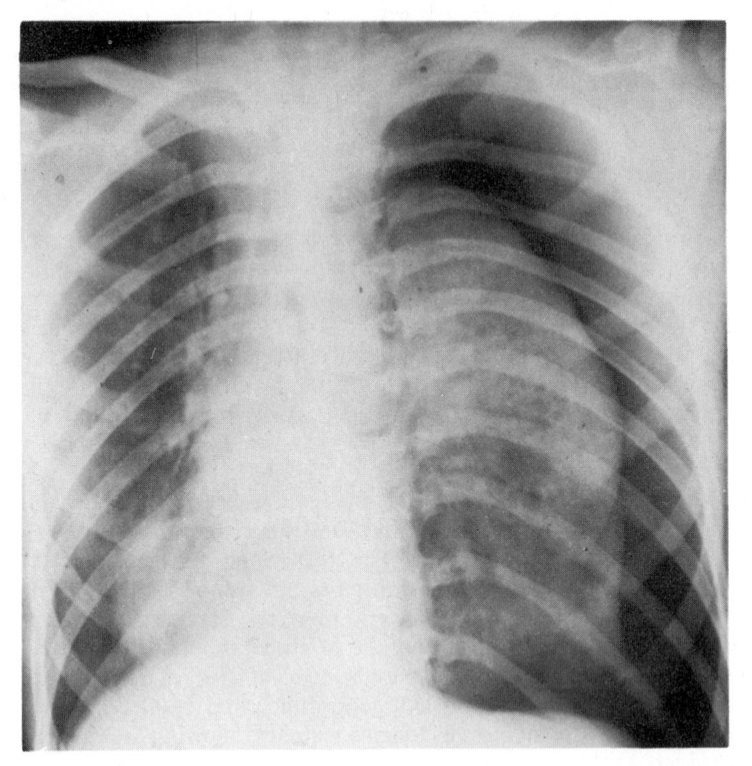

Fig. 33. Left tension pneumothorax associated with traumatic rupture of the left main bronchus.

of the chest wall and radiography showed persistent left pneumothorax. Bronchoscopy showed the left main bronchus to be plugged by blood clot and following its removal by suction, immediate and continued leakage of air occurred through the intercostal drainage tube.

Left thoracotomy was undertaken almost immediately. The mediastinal pleura was almost intact except for a small hole adjacent to the left main bronchus, air escaping in quantity through this opening. The mediastinal pleura was widely opened revealing that the left main bronchus was completely avulsed from the trachea at the level of the tracheobronchial junction, the gap being about 3 cm. There was no evidence of injury to the pulmonary vessels, aorta or diaphragm. The bronchus was rejoined to the trachea using interrupted stainless-steel sutures. The patient thereafter made an uneventful recovery.

2. A 28-year-old patient was admitted to the Brompton Hospital in 1955 complaining of chronic cough productive of purulent sputum. There was a history that at the age of 4 years she had been involved in a road traffic accident and had been admitted to Westminster Hospital. At that time she was noted to have subcutaneous emphysema. She spent 4 months in hospital but was eventually discharged. She was readmitted on several occasions in the subsequent few years for dilatation of a right main bronchial stricture. Up to the time of her last admission she had remained well and was living a fairly normal life. When examined there were no abnormal physical signs in the chest. However, her chest radiograph was bizarre (*Fig*. 34). Bronchography (*Fig*. 35) and bronchoscopy confirmed that the right main bronchus was totally strictured, the right pleural cavity containing the left upper lobe and the left pleural cavity containing the left lower lobe. The right bronchial stump was clearly seen. This patient, who suffered traumatic rupture of the right bronchus as a child, eventually tolerated this lesion and was reported as remaining well in 1965.

CLOSED RUPTURE OF THE TRACHEA

This injury has been only rarely reported for in most instances it is incompatible with life or associated injuries prove rapidly fatal.

CASE REPORT

Following a road traffic accident a young man was admitted to hospital with multiple but superficial lacerations. He was noted to have surgical emphysema of the neck and face, and radiologically mediastinal emphysema and a fracture of the right 4th rib were seen. A small pneumothorax was present bilaterally. He rapidly recovered and was discharged from hospital 3 days after admission. Eight days after the original accident he was admitted to hospital with rapidly progressive dyspnoea and wheezing and was noted to have severe inspiratory stridor. Bronchoscopy was undertaken and a tight stricture was noted 4 cm distal to the vocal cords with an eccentric lumen 5 mm in diameter. Tracheal resection was undertaken as an urgent procedure. At this operation the stricture was shown to correspond in level to the suprasternal notch. Approximately 2 cm of trachea were excised and primary suture undertaken, following which the patient made an uneventful recovery (*Fig*. 36).

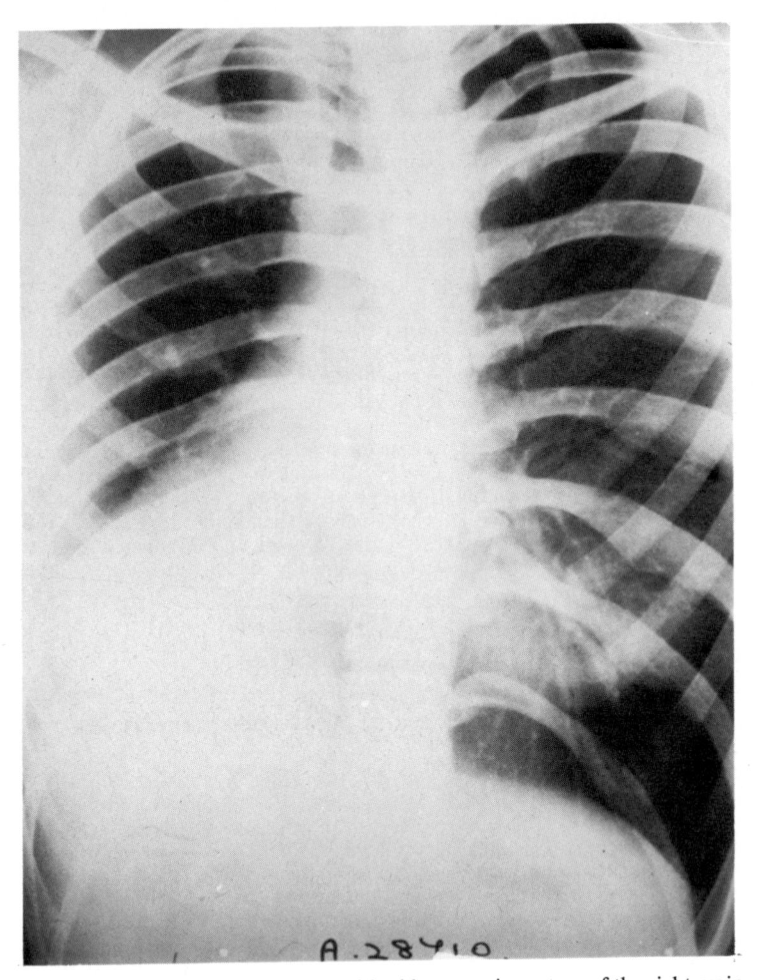

Fig. 34. Chest radiograph of patient with old traumatic rupture of the right main bronchus.

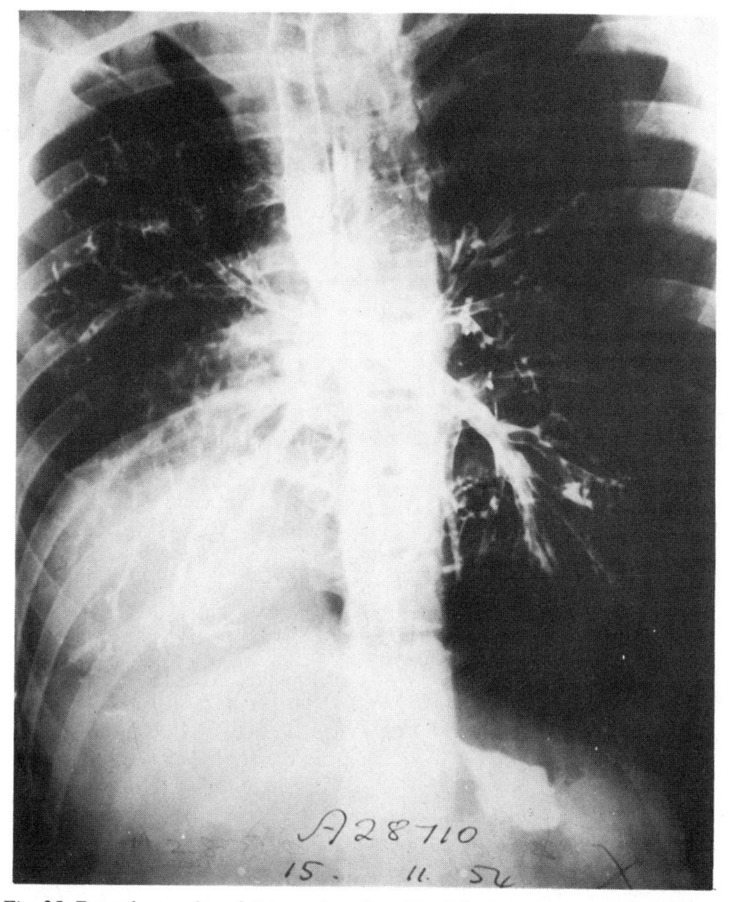

Fig. 35. Bronchography of this patient (*see Fig*. 34) demonstrates the left upper lobe to occupy the right chest and the left lower lobe to occupy the left chest.

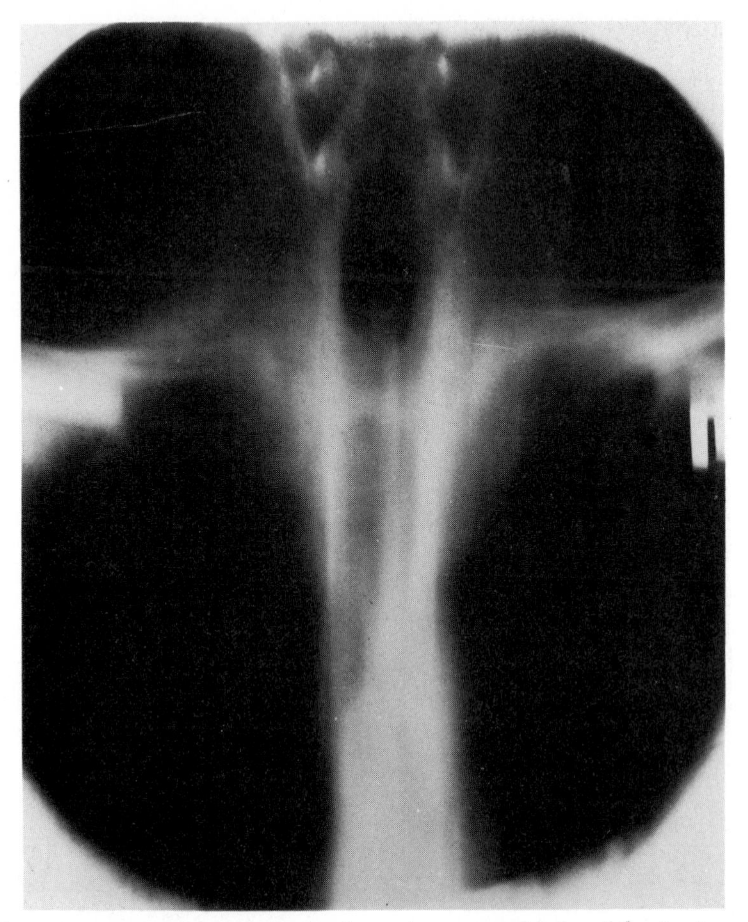

Fig. 36. Tomography of tracheal stricture demonstrated 8 days following traumatic rupture of the trachea. The nasogastric tube which appears to lie in the trachea is in fact in the oesophagus.

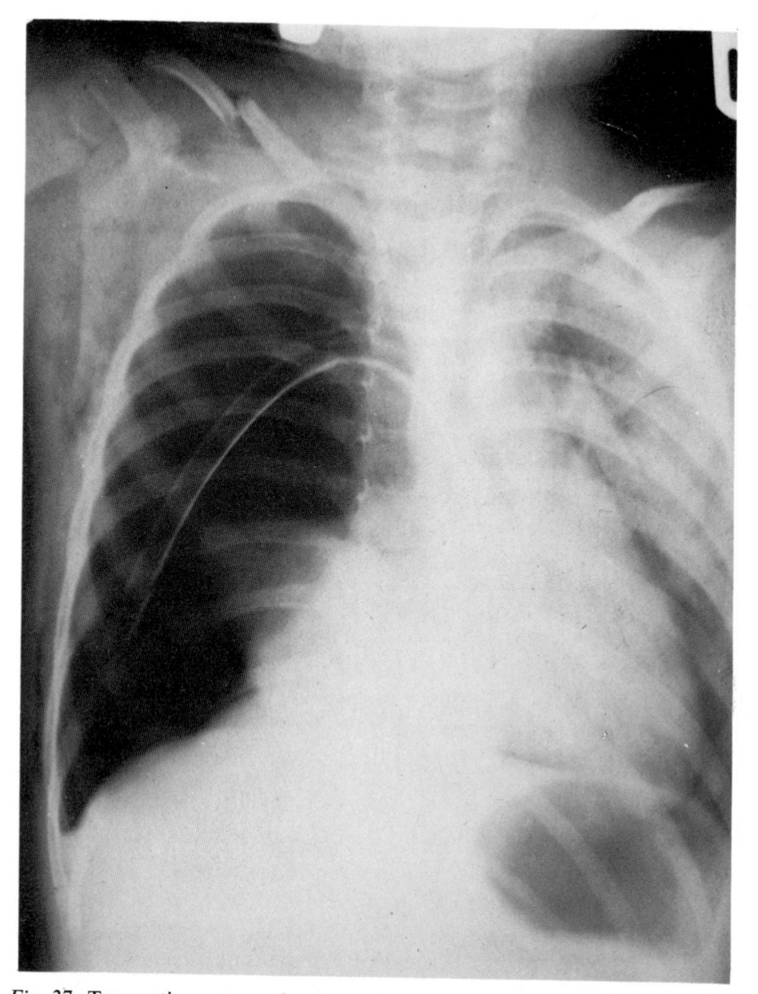

Fig. 37. Traumatic rupture of right main bronchus. The right lung appears to lie in the right cardiophrenic angle. At operation it was confirmed that the right main bronchus had completely separated and although the pulmonary vessels were intact the collapsed and airless lung lay on the diaphragm.

Chapter 11

Traumatic rupture of the diaphragm

The diagnosis of this injury is frequently delayed or completely missed since damage to the diaphragm is rarely an isolated injury and attention may be directed elsewhere. Closed rupture of the diaphragm is more usually associated with larger tears than those seen with penetrating and stab wounds, and may be accompanied by massive herniation of abdominal contents. Delay in diagnosis may cause severe respiratory embarrassment which is aggravated by general anaesthesia for the chest may fill with abdominal viscera which impairs ventilation. Should the diagnosis be missed, late strangulation of a previously unsuspected traumatic hernia may occur. From time to time patients present many years after an injury with a relatively symptom-free traumatic hernia.

CLOSED INJURIES (*see Fig.* 10)

Closed diaphragmatic rupture is associated with road traffic accidents or with falls from a height. Since there is no hernial sac, free passage of abdominal viscera into the chest may occur very early. The spleen is frequently lacerated and other serious chest, head and skeletal injuries are common. In the author's experience, 5 of his patients with ruptured diaphragm suffered associated rupture of the thoracic aorta. The patient may be shocked and dyspnoeic. The left hemithorax may be dull or hyperresonant and breath sounds may be replaced by bowel sounds, although bowel sounds are frequently inhibited at this stage by the associated ileus. As more bowel enters the chest the mediastinum may shift to the other side with development of a tension situation. In a few patients, however, symptoms and signs may be so vague that the diagnosis is overlooked. In these it is possible that a tear of the diaphragm may be plugged by abdominal viscera or omentum, with herniation occurring much later.

Diagnosis

Chest radiography in the erect position is diagnostic, as coils of bowel and stomach with fluid levels are seen. Occasionally herniated dilated stomach has been misdiagnosed as tension pneumothorax and treated by the introduction of an intercostal catheter. In these instances immediate clinical improvement is noted but the drainage of fluid for several days often causes consternation until it is noted to be gastric juice. From time to time confusion is caused by a localized lower thoracic pneumothorax which is trapped by lung adhesions. Elevation of the left diaphragm due to previous injury or even the large gas shadow of acute dilatation of the stomach has caused confusion (*see Fig.* 21). It should, however, rarely be necessary in recent herniation to undertake contrast radiology, and attempts at endoscopic diagnosis are not indicated.

Intrapericardial Rupture of Diaphragm

This is a rare injury. A tear produces free communication between the pericardial and abdominal cavities and if the tear extends into the pleuropericardium, the abdominal, pericardial and pleural cavities will be converted into one continuous chamber. This type of tear is not associated with cardiac herniation unless accompanied by a tear in the pleuropericardium. Its danger, however, lies in the tendency for upward herniation into the pericardial cavity of the abdominal viscera where incarceration or strangulation may occur. Clearly this lesion is accompanied by other major injuries and may therefore be overlooked.

Diagnosis

Radiologically, gas or bowel may be demonstrated within the pericardial cavity and from time to time barium contrast studies have demonstrated viscera within the pericardium. Of particular importance in this injury is the ease at which the diagnosis can be overlooked, even at thoracotomy. Robb (1963) described a patient who had been injured 23 years previously and in whom left thoracotomy showed no abnormality. A right thoracotomy was undertaken some months later when the stomach was observed through the right pleuropericardium and further exploration demonstrated the rent in the diaphragmatic pericardium.

Both rupture of pleuropericardium and of the diaphragmatic pericardium are rare but these lesions are far from benign and the possibility of such injuries should be borne in mind. Borrie and Lichter (1974) described 4 such cases and reviewed the literature on this subject.

TREATMENT OF RUPTURED DIAPHRAGM

A nasogastric tube should be passed as aspiration of the stomach will reduce the size of the hernia, making the patient more fit for anaesthesia.

Approach

Although general surgeons favour an abdominal approach to repair rupture of the diaphragm, the exposure is less satisfactory than that gained by thoracotomy. Should serious subdiaphragmatic damage be suspected a combined thoraco-abdominal approach is preferable to laparotomy especially in penetrating injuries. However, if traumatic rupture of the diaphragm is suspected to be the only injury, left thoracotomy through the 7th intercostal space is recommended. The herniated organs are examined, a torn or ruptured spleen is removed and injuries to the stomach and bowel, whether by penetration or strangulation, are appropriately dealt with. The hernia is then reduced. The tear usually radiates from the junction of the tendinous and muscular portions of the diaphragm, extending to but not including the crura. The tear is often linear and is repaired with two rows of continuous non-absorbable sutures, and the chest is closed with drainage. If further abdominal damage is suspected it is unwise to incise the diaphragm to facilitate inspection. Instead the thoracotomy incision should be extended across the left upper quadrant of the abdomen in an oblique manner.

CASE REPORTS

1. A 22-year-old girl was admitted to hospital following a road traffic accident in which she was the front seat passenger. A diagnosis of dislocation of the left hip was made which was reduced under general anaesthesia. Three days post-operatively the patient became extremely short of breath and cyanosed and a diagnosis of pulmonary embolism was entertained by the orthopaedic surgeons. Fortunately, a chest radiograph (the first since admission) clearly demonstrated a ruptured left leaf of the diaphragm. At operation there was a 15-cm tear from the dome of the diaphragm extending towards the oesophageal hiatus through which the stomach and much of the colon and small intestine had herniated (*see Fig*. 10, p. 33).

2. A man of 68 was referred by his doctor complaining of a history of shortness of breath which had recently become more severe. A recent chest radiograph had shown the lower half of the left chest to be occupied by gas and fluid levels. It was considered likely that the diaphragm was abnormally high in the chest, a condition sometimes known as 'eventration'. However, the patient gave a history of being involved in a motor vehicle accident 15 years earlier, and barium studies demonstrated the stomach to be inverted and high in the chest. At left thoracotomy there was found to be a hole 8 cm in diameter medial to the dome of the left diaphragm, through which had herniated stomach, small bowel and splenic flexure. These viscera were very adherent to the edges of the defect and to the lung.

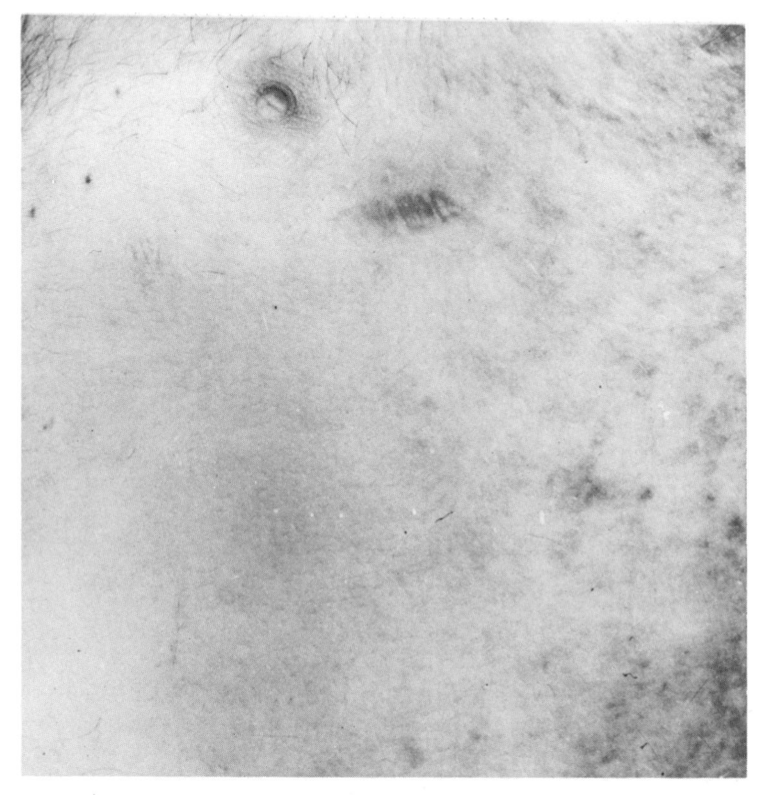

Fig. 38. Healed stab wound 3 cm below and to the left of the left nipple. The patient died, of strangulation of a loop of bowel by a traumatic diaphragmatic hernia resulting from this injury, 1 year later.

PENETRATING INJURIES

The diaphragm varies considerably in position depending on the phase of respiration. Consequently stab wounds of the chest may readily penetrate the diaphragm causing unsuspected serious sub-diaphragmatic damage (*see Fig*. 45, p. 126).

CASE REPORTS

1. A 19-year-old boy complained of severe and recurrent attacks of left chest pain and nausea. No chest radiograph was taken and no significance was attached to the history of a stab wound of the left chest 1 year earlier. There was a healed stab wound 2 cm long and 3 cm below and to the left of the left nipple. Development of severe chest pain, vomiting and profound collapse required his removal to hospital where he died shortly afterwards. At autopsy a loop of small bowel had entered the chest by way of a 2-cm hole in the diaphragm and had strangulated with perforation (*Fig*. 38).

2. A 35-year-old male patient was admitted who had been stabbed in the left side of the chest in the 8th intercostal space in the midaxillary line. The stab wound was 1·5 cm long. A left haemopneumothorax was drained using an intercostal catheter but despite adequate re-expansion of the lung and cessation of bleeding tachycardia persisted. There was no abdominal tenderness. In view of the site of the stab wound, the lower chest and abdomen were explored by an incision across the anterior end of the 7th intercostal space extending obliquely across the upper abdomen. The knife had penetrated the lower lobe of the left lung which had sealed, penetrated the left dome of diaphragm, transfixed the spleen, transfixed the splenic flexure of the colon and perforated the small intestine. There was considerable peritoneal soiling but, following splenectomy and repair of intestinal perforations, the patient recovered.

Gunshot wounds of the diaphragm may produce sufficient tissue destruction to render closure difficult. In such instances the diaphragm may be sutured higher to the chest wall. If closure is impossible it may be necessary to use a teflon or dacron prosthetic patch and in the absence of contamination such patches serve their purpose well.

Chapter 12

Traumatic chylothorax

Although chylothorax may complicate procedures such as Blalock anastomosis, ligation of patent ductus and oesophageal surgery, the reported incidence following closed or penetrating trauma is very low. It is, however, likely that chylothorax occurs more commonly than is appreciated and may account for some post-traumatic pleural effusions, which readily absorb and pass unnoticed. Closed rupture of the thoracic duct is associated with hyperextension of the spine, falls from a height or crush injuries. Characteristically recovery from the original injury is followed by a latent period of several days or weeks when the patient notices progressive shortness of breath on exertion. Dehydration and loss of weight may be a feature of this injury and at a late stage circulatory collapse may occur. Clinical and radiological examinations demonstrate a large pleural effusion and aspiration of milky fluid is diagnostic. However, in the early stages, and especially if the patient is not adequately fed, the fluid may be less milky in appearance. The presence of chyle is confirmed by examining the fluid microscopically and fat staining of the globules is positive. From time to time the site of rupture has been demonstrated by lymphangiography, when leakage of dye occurs very rapidly.

Since 80 per cent of ingested fat reaches the bloodstream by way of the thoracic duct, it is clear that the physiological consequences of rupture may be severe. Up to 2 litres of chyle daily are transported by the thoracic duct and the amount of fluid loss following injury may be quite serious.

Treatment

In the great majority of cases spontaneous closure of the thoracic duct will follow conservative measures. These consist of reduction of flow of chyle and removal of chyle from the chest. A low fat diet will often decrease chyle formation but in some patients intravenous feeding may be necessary. Repeated aspirations and intercostal drainage will enable the lung to expand. Surprisingly infection of chylothorax is extremely rare and this is attributed to the bacteriostatic effect of chyle.

Indications for Thoracotomy

Opinion is divided concerning the timing of operative intervention. The first successful operative intervention for a torn thoracic duct was described in 1948 by Lampson, and others later recommended that ligation of the thoracic duct be attempted if, despite aspiration and drainage for 2 weeks no improvement had occurred (Goorwich, 1955). More recently, however, opinion has again hardened in favour of a rather longer period of conservative management before thoracotomy is recommended (Maloney and Spencer, 1956; Williams and Burford, 1963). Despite many weeks of apparent unrelenting drainage of chyle and increasing gloom in the observers, cessation of flow is usually sudden and permanent in most patients. However, in the event of deterioration due to excessive loss of fluid, fat and electrolytes, or extreme deterioration in the patient's morale, operation should be undertaken after 3 weeks. The site of rupture may sometimes be demonstrated by lymphangiography. Operation should be preceded by the ingestion of 100 ml of cream 1 hour preoperatively which will encourage a profuse flow of chyle. Right thoracotomy is the exposure of choice and the mediastinum is explored in the region of the inferior vena cava. It is said that the site of leak is readily defined and in the author's experience of 1 case this was so. The leak requires suture ligation both above and below.

CASE REPORT

A middle-aged man was referred to hospital complaining of increasing shortness of breath. A chest X-ray demonstrated a large right pleural effusion. He gave a history of a fall from his bicycle 6 weeks earlier and although he remounted and rode away with no apparent injury his chest was very sore for some days. Chest aspiration was rewarded by the removal of 2 litres of milky fluid with re-expansion of the lung. Further aspirations were undertaken at 3- or 4-day intervals but at the end of 4 weeks there was no improvement and a total of 12 litres of chyle had been removed. Right thoracotomy was undertaken following the ingestion of a cream meal, and the leaking thoracic duct was readily identified immediately posterior to the inferior vena cava within the chest, where it was ligated. The patient recovered with no further pleural collection.

Chapter 13

Oesophageal injuries

Oesophageal injuries are serious as they frequently go unrecognized until a late stage when mediastinitis and pleural infection are established. Unless properly managed, these patients usually die slowly and miserably with multiple fistulae and drainage tubes and perhaps after several operations. Oesophageal injuries, either closed or open, are not common and if associated with trauma are usually one of many injuries which go unsuspected. However, instrumental perforations are by no means rare and if recognized early their mortality and morbidity are low. Unhappily, numerous endoscopic examinations of the oesophagus are undertaken by practitioners unfamiliar with either oesophageal surgery or indeed general surgery, and the gastro-enterologist, who is frequently not a surgeon, innocently passes rigid or flexible diagnostic instruments down the gullet in ever-increasing numbers. Unfortunately, the less experienced the endoscopist the more lightly he goes about his work and it is in such hands that serious delays are frequent. It must be recognized that even in expert hands oesophageal perforation can and does occur.

Experience has shown that symptoms of perforation that develop following discharge from hospital may go unheeded until a late stage. Since many oesophageal perforations will be caused by surgeons and physicians unskilled in their diagnosis and management and since this will often occur in centres where the immediate services of a thoracic surgeon are not available, it is inevitable that such perforations will be seen in the first instance by general surgeons who may themselves be unfamiliar with oesophageal surgery. It is hoped that the following advice will be useful.

At this stage it should be noted that an oesophageal perforation in many respects resembles an intestinal or particularly a colonic perforation in that there is rapid release of heavily infected contents into poorly supported tissues and spaces. Furthermore, like any intestinal perforation, oesophageal perforations will rarely close spontaneously and will rarely remain closed after suture in the presence of distal obstruction. Since many endoscopic examinations of the gullet and stomach are undertaken in the presence of such disease, it is clear that the treatment of such perforations must include treatment of the original disease, sometimes in circumstances of great disadvantage and in a contaminated surgical field. Thus perforations above a carcinoma or peptic stricture require emergency resection, and perforation above a hiatus hernia will require concomitant repair of the hernia.

INSTRUMENTAL PERFORATION

This may occur anywhere in the oesophagus but is more commonly seen in the cervical oesophagus or just above the diaphragm. Although such perforations are considered to be more common in elderly patients whose osteophytic projections on the cervical spine are said to compress the oesophageal wall against the instrument, this accident just as readily occurs in the young and mobile and may follow an apparently simple and uncomplicated investigation. The cause is more likely to be a combination of rough instrumentation, poor anaesthesia and bad luck, the last being the privilege of the expert, and perforation may occur using either the rigid or flexible instrument.

CERVICAL PERFORATIONS

Symptoms

Pain, tenderness, oedema and cervical subcutaneous emphysema are the cardinal signs of this injury and there may be an associated spike of temperature. Although some soreness may follow oesophagoscopy, pain and tenderness should be taken seriously. If undiagnosed para-oesophageal abscess may rapidly develop and be complicated by laryngo-pharyngeal oedema with respiratory obstruction.

Diagnosis

Gastrografin swallow is diagnostic. There is no place for demonstrating the perforation by further oesophagoscopy.

Management

A short period of conservative management using intravenous fluids and antibiotics is often successful, but unless clearly beneficial, operative exposure should not be long delayed. The oesophagus is exposed via an incision along the line of the anterior border of the sternomastoid muscle dissecting the plane of the strap muscles and elevating a lobe of the thyroid gland if necessary. The oedema fluid and thin pus form early. If seen, the tear is sutured with interrupted stainless-steel wire, but frequently a tear may not be seen. The wound is drained with soft latex. A feeding gastrostomy is undertaken and an intravenous infusion begun. Antibiotics are given. After 4 days small drinks are allowed and Gastrografin swallow repeated. All being well, the diet is gradually increased and the gastrostomy tube removed. A small fistula may persist for some weeks but is well sealed from the surrounding tissues and in the absence of distal obstruction usually dries rapidly.

THORACIC OESOPHAGEAL PERFORATION

Tears may occur in the mid-mediastinum but are more common just above the cardia. The pleura may initially remain intact permitting virulent mediastinal infection to track up and down but this soon ruptures into the pleura producing pyopneumothorax.

Symptoms

The patient complains of severe pain shortly after examination. The pain may be between the shoulder blades or in one or other side of the chest. Lateral chest pain or upper abdominal pain confirms pleural perforation and indicates the side. There is an associated temperature rise. Clinical and radiological examination may show little for up to 12 hours until pyopneumothorax occurs, although careful scrutiny of the mediastinum often shows early emphysema which may be palpated in the neck. A Gastrografin swallow is diagnostic. The clinical and radiological evidence of such perforations are not long delayed and the patient soon becomes very ill (*Figs*. 39, 40 *and see Fig*. 13*b*).

Treatment

Conservative treatment is misguided and operation is urgent. Delay of a few hours is permissible in order to replace fluids and electrolytes intravenously.

Thoracotomy is undertaken on the appropriate side. Despite the perhaps almost normal appearance of chest radiographs, a surprising

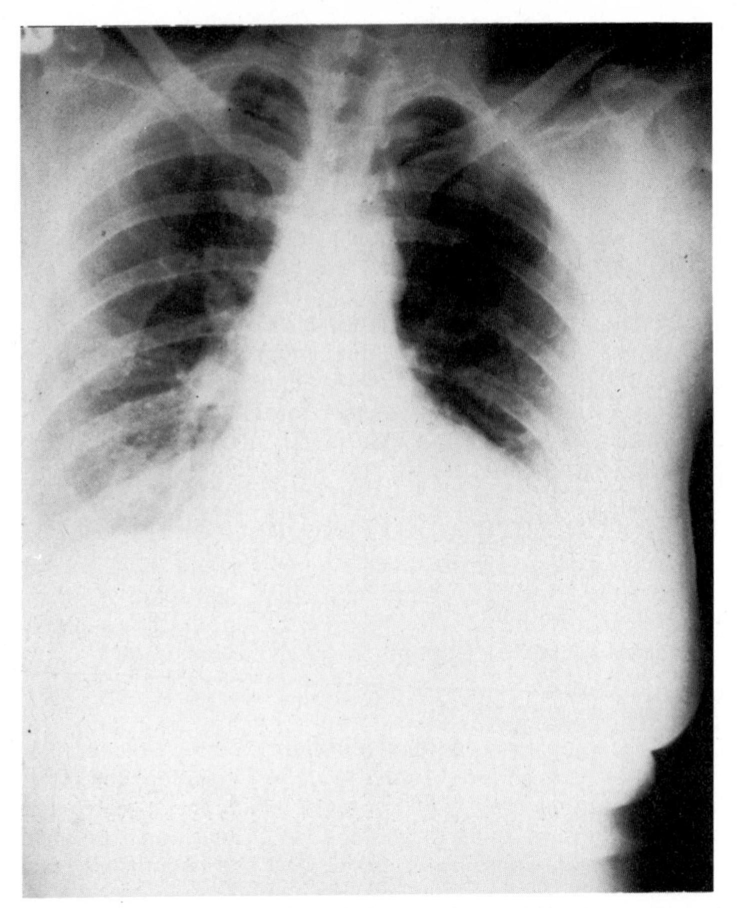

Fig. 39. Instrumental perforation of the oesophagus. This chest radiograph, which was taken 4 hours following oesophagoscopy and which demonstrates a small left pneumothorax, was passed as showing no abnormality.

amount of foul smelling, turbid fluid is invariably present in the pleural cavity, and the mediastinum is red, oedematous and contains many emphysematous bullae. It seems that in the presence of gastro-oesophageal reflux (for which the examination may have been undertaken) the refluxed gastric juice causes more serious damage and exudation than would otherwise be the case. The gullet is dissected out of its oedematous bed and the tear is usually readily seen. It is 2–3 cm long and is commonly just above the cardia where it is readily closed, or deep to the aortic arch where it is more

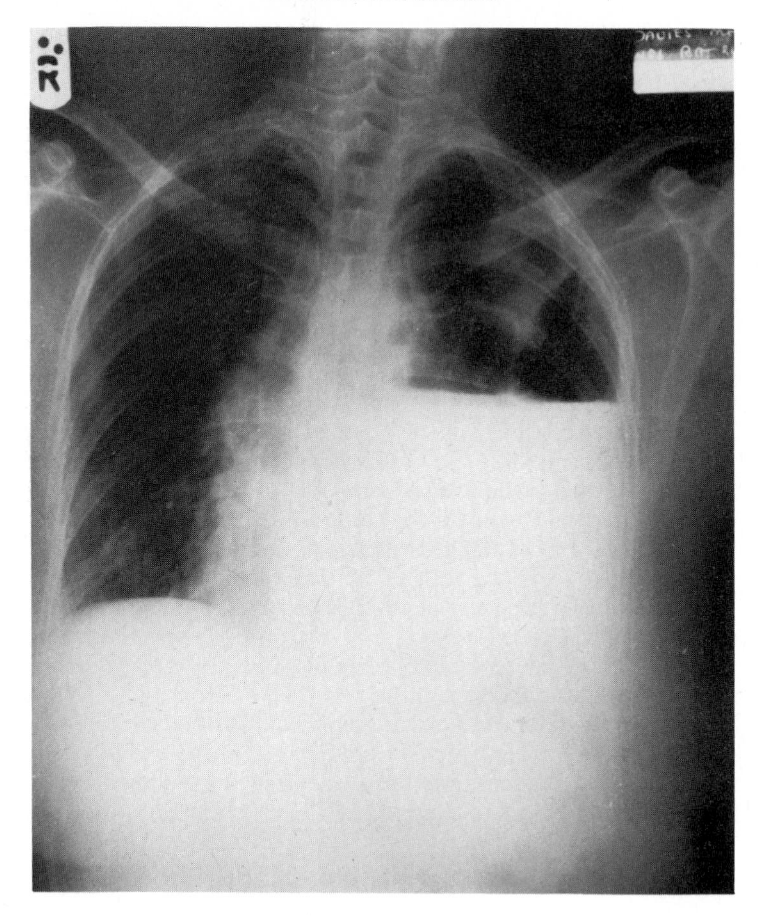

Fig. 40. The same patient as in *Fig.* 39. This chest radiograph was taken 24 hours following oesophagoscopy and now clearly demonstrates a large hydropneumothorax.

inaccessible. The edges are cleaned and sutured with interrupted fine stainless-steel wire sutures. The chest is closed with drainage.

The oesophagus is friable, and feeding gastrostomy or jejunostomy is desirable and is maintained for 14 days. Intravenous alimentation and antibiotics will also be required. In the majority of these patients the postoperative course is uncomplicated and Gastrografin swallow after 14 days is normal. However, in some patients an empyema will develop which may or may not be associated with further leakage. In the absence of a leak, the empyema is drained by closed followed by open drainage and healing is to be expected. If further leakage is demonstrated radiologically this will be confirmed by the appearance of ingested fluids, food or a test dose of dye appearing in the drainage bottle. The latter test, that of asking the patient to drink 10 ml of methylene blue, is almost diagnostic for in the presence of a leak it will invariably appear in the drainage bottle. If the leak is small gastrostomy feeding is continued and in many cases it will eventually close spontaneously. Further attempts to close the perforation at this stage are futile. If, however, the leak is severe loss of fluids may be serious. The fluids may be refluxed gastric juice and bile in addition to pleural inflammatory exudate. These fluid collections maintain large spaces within the pleura, and empyema formation in inevitable. Fluid loss is readily compounded by widespread intrathoracic infection, and in these patients toxaemia and septicaemia may be rapidly followed by death. In such patients it must be accepted that spontaneous cure is unlikely and that in the absence of radical treatment the battle will be lost.

The correct and courageous decision is that of emergency oesophagectomy. Experience teaches us that there is no place in the treatment of a large persistent oesophageal leak for the waiting-and-hoping régime (Keen, 1968). Early exploration is necessary and oesophagectomy offers the only hope of survival for these patients. Surgeons are naturally reluctant to remove the oesophagus, the more so if they caused the original instrumental perforation. Although oesophagectomy and subsequent oesophageal reconstruction is not entirely what the patient expected at the time of his admission for a 'minor' investigation, the alternative is less acceptable.

Operation

The chest is reopened and the oesophagus divided at the cardia which is closed and invaginated into the stomach. The oesophagus is separated from its attachments up to the first rib, and following removal of pus and fibrin from the chest and removal of peel from the lung, the chest is closed with drainage. The neck is explored and the oesophagus delivered. Much of this is removed and the remainder brought out into the posterior triangle of the neck as a cervical oesophagostomy. Its edges are sutured to the edge of a circular skin stoma away from the incision. Gastrostomy is undertaken.

The patient's condition rapidly improves and few are too ill to be denied the benefits of this life-saving procedure. Feeding gastrostomy is continued and the patient is allowed to recover from his experience. It is usually at least 8 weeks before oesophageal reconstruction can be considered. In younger patients colonic interposition is appropriate and it is the author's method of choice, using the left colon, splenic flexure and part of the transverse colon pedicled on the ascending branch of the left colic artery and vein. The graft is placed in the left chest and the operation undertaken in one stage (Belsey, 1965).

Others prefer subcutaneous or retrosternal interposition of the ascending colon. In the elderly or hypertensive, the mesocolic vasculature is unreliable and it is safer to elevate the stomach from the abdomen through the left chest and perform oesophagogastric anastomosis within the neck.

SPONTANEOUS RUPTURE OF THE OESOPHAGUS

This injury classically follows violent vomiting. The tear is often short and just above the cardia or may be larger extending to the aortic arch. In some instances the oesophagus has several large tears giving the impression of an internal explosion which may, in fact, represent the aetiology. It is believed that this accident is caused by incoordination of the vomiting reflexes. During vomiting, as the stomach strongly contracts, the oesophagus and its upper sphincter normally relax allowing unimpeded ejection of gastric contents. Should the cricopharyngeal sphincter contract at the same time as does the stomach, the huge pressure build-up in the gullet may rupture it where it is least supported. Surprisingly enough, vomiting with a nasogastric tube in the oesophagus affords no protection and the author has experience of 2 patients sustaining such ruptures several days after routine abdominal operations, following vomiting, and in both the rupture was massive. This injury was apparently common in bygone days of serious eating and was first described by Boerhaave in 1724. The first report of successful repair was by Barrett in 1946.

Symptoms

These are characteristic. Shortly after a very large meal or the ingestion of a considerable amount of fluid (often alcoholic) violent vomiting occurs which is quickly followed by sudden and agonizing chest pain, although from time to time pain is in the epigastrium which may confuse the diagnosis. The patient soon becomes shocked and is clearly very ill. At this stage a diagnosis of myocardial infarction, acute pancreatitis or perforated duodenal ulcer is common and understandable. However, chest examination should disclose evidence of air and fluid in the chest, usually on the left side. If a routine chest radiograph is taken on all patients with severe chest pain or upper abdominal pain, this injury would be misdiagnosed less frequently. Gastrografin swallow will confirm the diagnosis and identify the site and side of rupture.

Treatment

Although on rare occasions patients may be seen at a late stage with an empyema consequent on such perforation and who respond to empyema drainage, the great majority will die in the absence of surgical closure and operation is advised. The appropriate side of the chest is opened. The appearance is similar to that described for instrumental perforation although in this case the pleural cavity is soiled by undigested food or alcoholic beverages. If the tear is short it is closed with interrupted stainless-steel wire sutures and gastrostomy performed. The subsequent treatment is similar to that of instrumental perforation. If the gullet has exploded and has torn at several sites simple suture will be inevitably followed by further breakdown. In these patients oesophagectomy, gastrostomy and oesophagostomy are necessary to save the patient and later oesophageal reconstruction will follow.

EXTERNAL BLUNT TRAUMA

The oesophagus may very rarely be damaged in closed injuries, and usually in association with deceleration against a car steering wheel. The mechanism is that of nipping of the trachea and oesophagus in the upper thorax between the manubrium sterni and the vertebral bodies. This is therefore an injury of the young whose elastic ribs will allow such compression and recoil. There are usually other associated injuries and oesophageal damage will often be overlooked. However, the presence of subcutaneous emphysema in the neck and hydropneumothorax should prompt examination of the oesophagus by means of Gastrografin radiography. If a tear is demonstrated, early exploration is advised. From time to time such injuries may cause traumatic tracheo-oesophageal fistula producing ready inhalation of food and fluids, and its presence is confirmed by contrast radiography (*see Figs.* 13*a* and 16). These injuries are sometimes amenable to direct closure but the damage is often so severe that oesophagectomy followed by oesophageal reconstruction is inevitable (Overstreet and Ochsner, 1955; Worman et al., 1962; Michelson and Roque, 1968).

PENETRATING OESOPHAGEAL INJURIES

The oesophagus may be injured within the neck or chest by gunshot or other penetrating injuries. The diagnosis should be made at the time of exploration for any such injury which could conceivably have injured the gullet should be explored. Simple tears may be sutured but again damage is often extensive, precluding such repair and requiring delayed reconstruction.

OESOPHAGEAL INJURIES PRODUCED BY FOREIGN BODIES

Although this injury is usually associated with endoscopic removal of the foreign body, foreign bodies may from time to time spontaneously penetrate the wall of the oesophagus. Particularly dangerous in this respect are fragments of chicken or rabbit bone, or dental plates. These objects are usually radiotranslucent and their presence difficult to detect. The patient's history is typical. Several days or perhaps as long as 2 weeks following a choking episode whilst eating, massive haematemesis may be followed by the rapid death of the patient but more frequently there are several less serious episodes of haematemesis followed inevitably by a final massive haemorrhage. At autopsy the bone is seen to lie in an abscess between the oesophagus and thoracic aorta penetrating both structures. Such a catastrophe was happily avoided in the case of the following patient.

CASE REPORT

A 15-year-old boy swallowed an upper denture while playing cricket in August 1967. He was admitted to his local hospital where radiography failed to demonstrate the presence of a foreign body. However, oesophagoscopy was undertaken there on the day of admission and again 4 days later but no denture was seen. Gastrotomy was performed with a negative result. Eight days after his accident he became very ill with clinical and radiological evidence of left pyopneumothorax and he was transferred to the thoracic unit. Gastrografin swallow showed the negative shadow of the denture at the lower end of the oesophagus but no leak was detected.

Left thoracotomy was undertaken on the same day. There was a large empyema. At the lower end of the oesophagus there was an abscess bounded anteriorly by the pericardium, posteriorly by the aorta and inferiorly by the diaphragm. The lung was firmly adherent to the abscess at this level. It was necessary to peel the lung from the oesophagus, reopening a ragged hole at its lower end, through which the jagged palatal part of the dental plate was protruding and pressing against the lower end of the thoracic aorta. The foreign body was removed; there was no hope of closing the oesophagus at this stage. Since the lung had originally closed this oesophageal fistula it was considered that it would do so again with a little help. The left lower lobe of the lung was therefore decorticated and sutured to the edges of the oesophageal defect with interrupted catgut sutures and the pleural cavity was drained.

Feeding gastrostomy was performed, and was used for 21 days and no fluids were given by mouth. A Gastrografin swallow at this stage showed a normal-appearing oesophagus with no evidence of leak. Feeding by mouth was gradually instituted and the gastrostomy tube was removed after another week, with an uninterrupted recovery. Barium swallow 6 weeks later showed no oesophageal abnormality. The patient is well 17 years later and has no symptoms.

Chapter 14

Closed injuries of the heart and pericardium

The heart and pericardium may be injured by closed or penetrating trauma; severe injuries are not necessarily incompatible with life. Those who reach hospital alive frequently do so because cardiac tamponade prevents massive haemorrhage and with prompt surgery many such patients survive. The heart is a robust organ and as long as the main coronary vessels are undamaged and adequately perfused with oxygenated blood it will beat faithfully (Naclereo, 1964).

PERICARDIAL INJURIES

The pericardium may be torn following closed trauma but such tears are less important than the underlying cardiac damage, which may be severe (Guest et al., 1965). *See* p. 93.

RUPTURED PLEUROPERICARDIUM

This is by far the more common injury and the tear is usually vertical and may communicate with the right or left pleural cavity. The tear may be small but if of more than moderate size, part or the whole of the heart may herniate. If the herniation is restricted to an atrial appendage the function of the heart will not be impaired. If, however, the tear is larger the heart may herniate entirely from the pericardial cavity into the pleural cavity and suffer gross impairment of its action.

Diagnosis

Although pericardial rupture will accompany the injury, cardiac herniation may be delayed for several days. An unusual heart outline seen on initial or later chest radiographs may suggest the diagnosis. Cine-angiography may confirm the diagnosis but the condition may cause such severe symptoms that there may be little time for such investigations. The effects of rupture of the pleuropericardium closely parallel those of congenital absence of the pericardium (Borrie, 1969). Boxall, in 1886, described the fatal escape of the heart into the left pleural cavity following trauma.

Treatment

Should the diagnosis be suspected, immediate thoracotomy on the appropriate side is advised. Small tears may be readily sutured but larger rents, especially of some days' duration, may be impossible to close and in these situations a patch of woven Dacron should be sutured to the edges of the defect preventing herniation.

CARDIAC INJURIES

Closed damage to the heart may be caused by steering wheel injuries and varies in severity from contusion to rupture of the organ. Falls from a height may avulse the heart from the aortic root, and the extreme deceleration of aircraft accidents is a prominent cause of cardiac damage.

MYOCARDIAL CONTUSIONS

These are usually of less significance than associated injuries, for the energy required to bruise the heart is usually accompanied by severe trauma locally and elsewhere. The contusions vary from petechial haemorrhages beneath the epicardium to large deep areas of intramuscular bruising and bleeding. Such damaged areas may progress to softening and delayed rupture.

Diagnosis

The patient may complain of retrosternal pain but more specific signs are unexplained tachycardia and palpitations. A friction rub may be heard after several days. In those with extensive muscle injury, shortness of breath or even pulmonary oedema may occur. Shortly after injury radiological evidence of cardiac enlargement is rare but pulmonary venous congestion or pulmonary oedema may be noted on the radiograph.

However, the electrocardiogram and estimation of enzyme levels offer the most reliable evidence of cardiac muscle damage. Typically, the ECG varies from patient to patient and from time to time in the same patient. Commonly, alterations in the ST segment suggestive of anoxia and widening of the QRS complex may be noted and varying degrees of heart block may suggest septal or nodal damage. Serum aspartate aminotransferase (SAAT) levels may be raised but such information will not be available during the first 24 hours. In older patients, the features of chest pain, ECG abnormalities and serum enzyme changes may sometimes cause difficulty in deciding whether the injury caused a myocardial contusion, or whether a myocardial infarct caused the patient to have his accident, and this may be of legal importance.

Treatment

No specific treatment is indicated but careful observation should be maintained, for from time to time cardiac tamponade may be associated with myocardial contusion. This may be difficult to differentiate from acute heart failure although pulmonary oedema is more likely to be associated with heart failure than is cardiac tamponade. When in doubt, careful pericardiocentesis may be of assistance.

If clinically and electrocardiographically severe, myocardial contusions may behave in a similar fashion to myocardial infarcts and produce arrhythmias, heart failure, late cardiac rupture or chronic aneurysm. Bed-rest for 2 weeks is indicated and general anaesthesia should be avoided if possible.

The ECG should be monitored and arrhythmias noted. Whereas these are usually of no serious significance frequent ventricular ectopic beats or bursts of ventricular tachycardia may give warning of impending ventricular fibrillation and with these patients it is wise to administer an anti-arrhythmic drug. Intravenous lignocaine hydrochloride in an initial dose of 1 mg per kg body weight followed by 1 mg per minute will usually abolish many or most of these abnormal complexes and this drug should be continued until a safer ECG is noted, following which the amount may be gradually reduced.

Delayed cardiac rupture is hardly a surgical problem but chronic ventricular aneurysm is amenable to accurate diagnosis and treatment.

CLOSED CARDIAC RUPTURE

This is frequently seen in fatal accidents, where the right ventricle is more often involved. Closed atrial rupture is rare but is compatible with longer survival, and a handful of such patients have survived early thoracotomy and repair of the torn chamber.

CLOSED RUPTURE OF THE INTERVENTRICULAR SEPTUM

This may occur at the time of injury or be delayed following necrosis of a septal contusion. When septal rupture is the sole injury, immediate survival is usual although cardiac failure may develop, for adaptation to this acute situation is poor. A tell-tale systolic murmur will encourage full investigation and should the shunt be large consideration should be given to surgical closure using cardiopulmonary by-pass. Small defects may close spontaneously and if the patient's condition is satisfactory a delay of several months is justified. Not only may the defect close in this time but should surgery be required the edges of the defect will have developed good fibrous tissue suitable for holding sutures (Guilfoil and Doyle, 1953; Pierce et al., 1958).

CLOSED INJURY TO THE HEART VALVES

Closed rupture of the heart valves is rarely compatible with survival but from time to time this injury is encountered, the aortic valve being most frequently and the pulmonary valve least commonly affected. Damage to the mitral and tricuspid valves is more usually that of chordal or papillary muscle rupture than of leaflet damage and may be caused by sudden and severe compression of the ventricles during systole. Aortic and mitral valve damage are invariably associated with severe congestive heart failure with pulmonary oedema, although on rare occasions patients may adapt to these injuries. Surprisingly, traumatic rupture of the tricuspid valve may be well tolerated for many years (Robin et al., 1974).

These patients commonly present with other major injuries and develop cardiac failure after a period of several days. Initially, intensive medical treatment including bed-rest, digoxin and diuretic therapy will be necessary and at this stage a cardiologist and cardiac surgeon may be consulted. It is wise to undertake cardiac catheterization early for later sudden deterioration may require urgent surgery. If despite treatment of heart failure the patient loses ground, surgical treatment using cardiopulmonary by-pass will be required and it is invariably necessary to replace the damaged valve or valves with either a prosthetic or biological substitute.

CASE REPORTS

1. A 57-year-old female patient was admitted, having been the front seat passenger in a motorcar that was involved in a road traffic accident. Within 2 days of admission she developed progressive and severe shortness of breath which was associated with the clinical and radiological signs of pulmonary

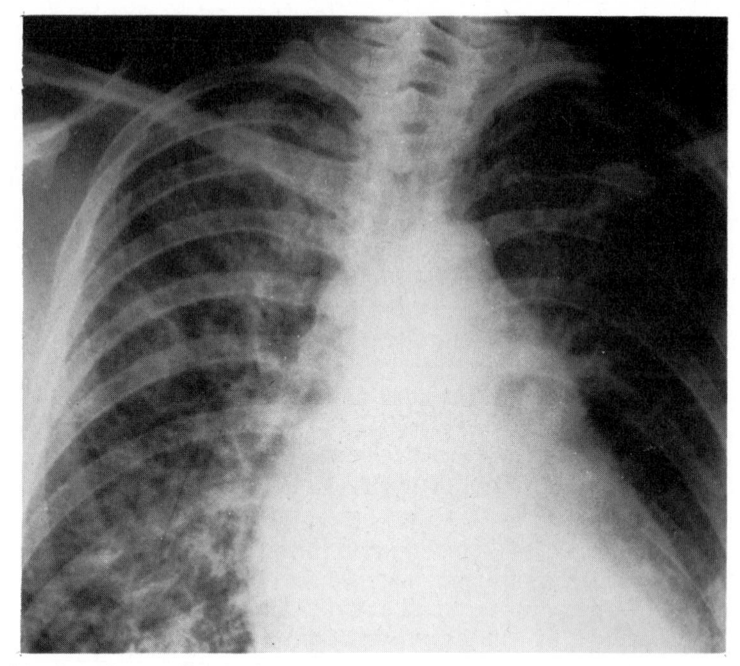

Fig. 41. Chest radiograph demonstrating pulmonary oedema. This patient developed acute traumatic mitral incompetence following a chest injury.

oedema. An apical systolic murmur was noted and she developed congestive heart failure. Cardiac catheterization and left ventricular cine-angiography confirmed the clinical impression of traumatic mitral incompetence. The patient responded well to intensive treatment with digoxin and diuretics and within a few weeks appeared to have compensated adequately for this disability. At the time of discharge the patient was well although the physical signs of free mitral incompetence were present. It was considered that mitral valve replacement would eventually be required, but the patient preferred that surgery be delayed as long as she remained apparently well (*Figs*. 41 and 42).

2. A 41-year-old man was transferred from another hospital 2 days following a road traffic accident in which he sustained multiple fractures and a chest injury. He became progressively short of breath and a systolic murmur was readily heard over the left precordium. When examined, there was marked venous pulsation in the neck and the liver was enlarged and pulsatile. Radiologically, pulmonary oedema was present and a clinical diagnosis of traumatic rupture of the mitral and tricuspid valves was confirmed at cardiac catheterization and angiography. Despite intensive medical treatment the patient's condition deteriorated and surgical operation was required using cardiopulmonary by-pass.

At operation the posterior cusp of the mitral valve was flail, all of its chordal attachments being ruptured, and there was furthermore a large rent in the anterior cusp of the mitral valve. The septal leaflet of the tricuspid valve was avulsed

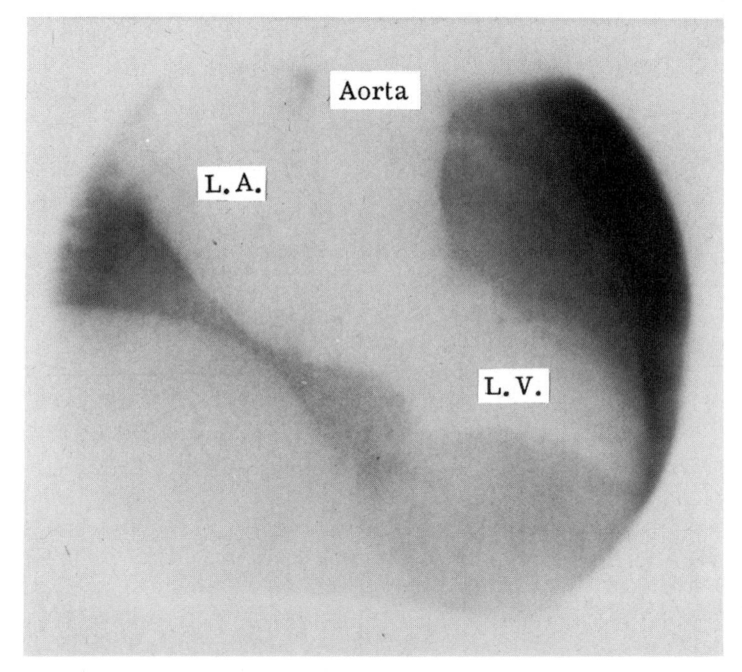

Fig. 42. Left ventricular cine-angiocardiogram of a patient demonstrating severe mitral incompetence. (*See Fig.* 41.)

from its chordal connections and the lateral leaflet of this valve was torn. Each valve was replaced with a Björck–Shiley disc valve. Despite immediate post-operative improvement the patient's condition deteriorated and he died in uraemic coma 10 days after his injury from peritonitis associated with unsuspected avulsion of the head of the pancreas and rupture of the duodenum.

CONSTRICTIVE PERICARDITIS

A rare consequence of either open or closed cardiac injuries is the late development of constrictive pericarditis. Although in the majority of patients haemopericardium is absorbed and the consequent fusion of pericardial layers is without ill effect, for some unexplained reason the reaction of others to haemopericardium is to proceed to pericardial constriction.

The features of this disease are similar to those of 'idiopathic' constrictive pericarditis or tuberculous constrictive pericarditis but the development of this condition within a few months or years of severe chest trauma may point to its aetiology. The treatment of this condition is pericardiectomy.

Chapter 15

Penetrating wounds of the heart and great vessels

Penetrating wounds of the chest and heart have attracted the attention of surgeons since the earliest times, but it was Rehn who described the first successful suture of a stab wound of the heart (Rehn, 1897). In 1907 he reported a large series of cardiac injuries managed surgically with a remarkably high survival rate (Rehn, 1907). Seventy years and many major wars later the outlook for patients with penetrating cardiac wounds has progressively improved, and since World War II pericardiocentesis has given way more and more to operative treatment. Hospitals in areas served by good communications can expect to admit patients very shortly after injury who formerly would have arrived dead. Such patients may require thoracotomy immediately and anaesthesia may be either unavailable or inadequate. However, such operations are frequently successful even in those with actual or imminent cardiac arrest, and in the presence of such an emergency the surgeon on the spot has little alternative but to proceed single handed. A skilled team, adequately supported with equipment and the facilities for rapid fluid and blood replacement, can expect surprisingly good results in this group of patients (Mattox et al., 1974).

An analysis of several large series describing patients with all types of penetrating cardiac wounds reveals that between 62 and 84 per cent die before reaching hospital, and the majority of these have suffered gunshot wounds (Mattox et al., 1974). On the other hand, the mortality rate from stab wounds of the heart varies between nil (Hardy and Williams, 1967) to 37·5 per cent (Steichen et al., 1971).

The great majority of heart wounds of surgical importance are therefore caused by knives and other sharp weapons. (Gunshot wounds are usually fatal before admission to hospital.) The type of wound varies and includes superficial nicks, penetration of the muscle, perforation into one or other chamber or transfixion of the heart. Solitary pericardial wounds account for less than 10 per cent of such injuries. Wounds of the ventricle account for 70 per cent of cardiac injuries, the anterior right ventricle being more commonly injured than the left although left ventricular stab wounds are less likely to reach hospital. Atrial wounds account for 10 per cent of injuries and solitary wounds of the pericardium, coronary arteries, ascending aorta, pulmonary artery and great veins account for the remainder. Any chest wound, either anteriorly or posteriorly situated, should alert the surgeon to the possibility of cardiac injury, as should any upper abdominal or subcostal stab wound. Ventricular aneurysm may present clinically months or years after stab wounds (Lyons and Perkins, 1958).

PERICARDIAL TAMPONADE

Although sometimes associated with blunt trauma, pericardial tamponade is usually caused by penetrating wounds.

Physiology of Pericardial Tamponade

Escape of blood from the heart into the pericardium causes compression unless the blood escapes either externally or into the pleural cavity. The mechanism of tamponade is more readily understood if the pericardium is considered as a bag incapable of rapid stretching. Escaping blood and blood clot will occupy the potential space between the heart and pericardium and compress the heart. It is, however, not so much compression which produces the disturbance as the associated interference with diastolic filling of the heart. For the heart to eject an adequate stroke volume it requires adequate space in which to relax and dilate during diastolic filling. Should the confines of the pericardial sac be partly occupied by blood clot, less room is available for diastolic filling with consequent diminution of stroke volume and cardiac output. Initially, increase in heart rate will compensate for the fall in cardiac output but should bleeding continue failure of forward flow with build up on the venous side will occur. As the right ventricle has a much lower pressure than the left, right ventricular obstruction will occur sooner than on the left side and a point will be reached at which cardiac output falls to such a low level that anoxic cardiac arrest will follow.

Physical Signs of Pericardial Tamponade

The cardinal signs are:

1. Fall in arterial pressure.
2. Rise in venous pressure.
3. Muffled heart sounds.
4. Paradoxical pulse.

It must be borne in mind that these signs may be difficult to elicit or be frankly misleading. Thus, distended neck veins or a rise in central venous pressure may not be noted if serious blood loss is associated with other injuries. On the other hand, straining and coughing may well be responsible for a raised venous pressure. Left tension pneumothorax classically mimics cardiac tamponade with distended neck veins and absent heart sounds in the left chest. Furthermore, listening for muffled heart sounds in a noisy admission ward may not be easy. The patient may appear cyanosed and in extreme cases venous congestion of the head, face and neck is prominent. The pulse is rapid and of low volume and the phenomenon of paradoxical pulsation may be readily demonstrated. Normally the pulse volume increases with inspiration, but in pericardial tamponade the already embarrassed right ventricle cannot cope with the extra venous return of inspiration and there is a consequent fall in cardiac output at this time. Another explanation offered is that of the tensing of the diaphragm by its downward pull during inspiration which further compresses the right ventricle. A decrease in systolic pressure greater than 15 mmHg during inspiration is highly suggestive of tamponade. The cardiac silhouette may be increased in size radiologically although serial films may be necessary to demonstrate this (*Fig*. 43). As heart action becomes less powerful the electrocardiographic voltage may be reduced. Haemothorax may be present if there is free passage from the pericardium to the pleural cavity but even under these circumstances tamponade may occur (*Fig*. 44).

Treatment

The diagnosis of pericardial tamponade should not await obvious and florid presentation of all physical signs for at this stage the patient may be but a short step from cardiac arrest. The nature of the injury should encourage close watch for development of these signs and the fully developed picture should be anticipated and treated.

Aspiration readily relieves tamponade, for the removal of as little as 20 ml of blood enables adequate diastolic filling to take place, restoring cardiac output. Furthermore, pericardiocentesis is a useful confirmatory test of traumatic haemopericardium. Despite great care and experience a heart chamber may be penetrated during this operation and the aspiration of blood may cause confusion.

Pericardiocentesis

Although both parasternal and subxiphoid routes have their advocates the subxiphoid is probably safer and more efficient. This should be performed in an operating theatre excepting under extremely critical conditions. Apart from the distinct possibility of cardiac arrest following unrelieved tamponade, the dangers of coronary vessel damage or the precipitation of a dangerous arrhythmia are real enough to require that this be undertaken with facilities for immediate thoracotomy at hand. ECG monitoring is strongly urged and the external defibrillator must be available at the bedside.

The patient should be sat up at 45°. The skin is sterilized and a cutaneous weal raised with local anaesthetic at the chosen site which is the angle between the xiphoid process and the left costal margin, following which local anaesthetic should be infiltrated to the pericardium. An 8-cm long medium bore needle is inserted upwards and backwards at an angle of 45° to the skin surface and directed 20° to the patient's left. At about 5 cm from the skin surface the pericardium is entered and although this is usually not palpable the characteristic feel of the heart beating or scraping on the needle point is unmistakable. Aspiration of blood will be rewarded by an improvement in the patient's condition. If ECG rhythm disturbances are noted, the needle should be withdrawn gradually until the arrhythmia terminates (Ravitch and Blalock, 1949; Elkin and Campbell, 1951).

Emergency Thoracotomy for Pericardial Tamponade

Instruments for thoracotomy must be available near the bedside of patients who are suspected of heart injury or are being treated by pericardial aspiration and in the event of severe hypotension or cardiac arrest immediate thoracotomy should be undertaken. The patient should be intubated and ventilated by an anaesthetist.

An incision is made from the left sternal edge to the anterior axillary line following the curve of the 5th rib and is rapidly deepened through the muscles of the chest wall until the ribs are exposed. The 4th intercostal space is entered and rapidly opened from end to end, protecting the underlying lung and clamping the internal mammary vessels. A simple self-retaining retractor or an assistant with a hook retractor under the upper edge of the rib cage will readily open the chest, or exposure may be improved by division of the costal cartilage of the upper rib. The tense, blue pericardium confirms the diagnosis

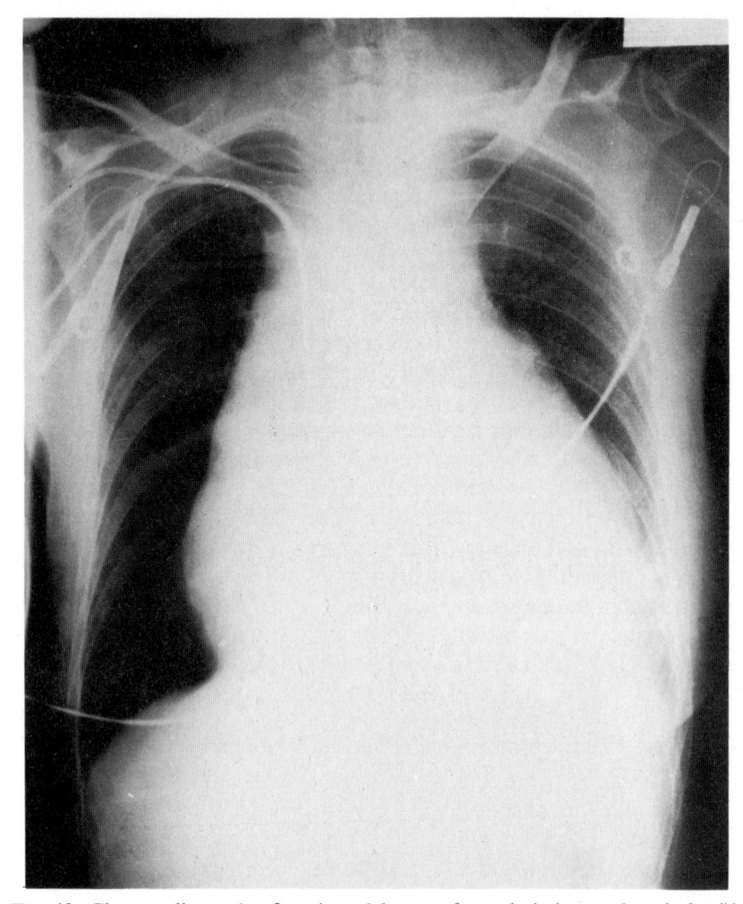

Fig. 43. Chest radiograph of patient 6 hours after admission to hospital with an epigastric stab wound. The heart shadow is considerably enlarged. At operation 800 ml of clot were removed.

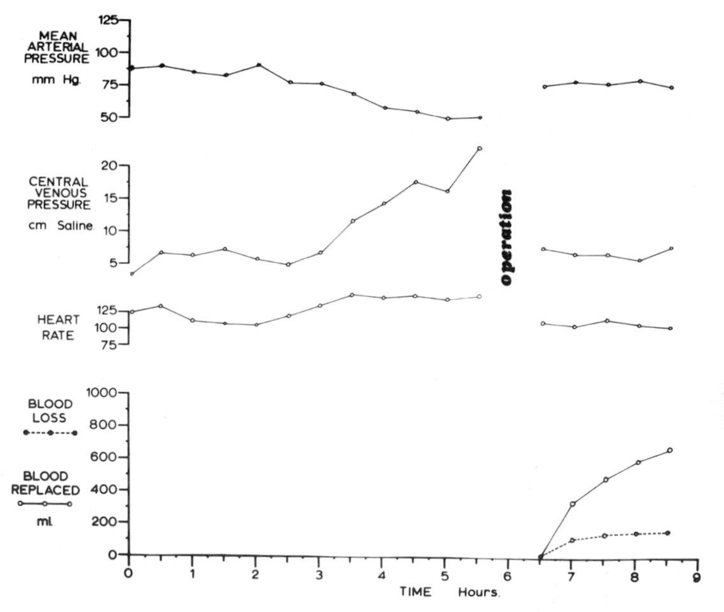

Fig. 44. Progress chart of patient shown in *Fig*. 43. The progressive fall in arterial pressure was accompanied by a rise in central venous pressure, and following evacuation of clot from the pericardium the arterial pressure rose and was accompanied by a fall in venous pressure to normal levels.

and blood clot or liquid exuding through a pericardial tear may define the site of myocardial injury. The pericardium is then picked up with forceps and opened with scissors anterior to the phrenic nerve, from the diaphragm up towards the pulmonary artery.

The release of clot and fluid blood is usually followed by a rapid improvement in cardiac action and output. The stab wound of the heart may be readily seen and, if spurting blood, is readily controlled by simple finger compression. Laceration of an atrial appendage may be controlled by a finger and thumb or a light non-crushing clamp. Cardiac wounds are readily repaired with interrupted or continuous non-absorbable sutures mounted on atraumatic needles, and a bleeding atrial appendage may be tied off below the controlling clamp or sutured. Bleeding coronary vessels are probably of no great consequence for damage to important vessels is not compatible with survival. Should bleeding persist, the apex of the heart may be gently elevated to expose the inferior and posterior surfaces, for from time to time a fully penetrating knife wound will perforate the heart posteriorly. Bleeding originating from the right atrium or the great veins may require division of the sternum and opening of the corresponding intercostal space on the right side in order to gain safe access. Cardiopulmonary by-pass is rarely necessary.

Penetrating damage to the septa or valves is clearly not amenable to treatment at this stage unless a cardiac surgical team is immediately available. However, it is fortunate that the patient who has survived pericardial tamponade is likely to tolerate complicated injuries long enough for full evaluation and treatment to be conducted at greater leisure. The pericardium is closed with three or four interrupted sutures and before closing the chest with drainage the internal mammary vessels are ligated and other bleeding points dealt with.

THE GENERAL MANAGEMENT OF STAB WOUNDS OF THE HEART AND GREAT VESSELS

Since many such wounds are self-sealing and respond to one or two pericardial aspirations, it has become the practice of some hospitals in the centre of large cities accustomed to extreme violence (notably in North America and South Africa) to avoid thoracotomy if possible in such patients. In the accident rooms of these hospitals patients with such stab wounds are so common that the staff and facilities to enable exploratory thoracotomy in all cases are not available. This policy has the merit of expedience and by and large in such centres few mistakes are made. It must, however, be made clear that such staff, in dealing with so great a number of stab wounds, develop a higher degree of skill and experience in the management of these injuries than is available elsewhere. In this country, stab wounds of the heart are comparatively rare and few surgeons have the appropriate experience which enables them to determine which are best treated by observation and aspiration and which by exploration.

For this reason a policy of exploration of all stab wounds of the heart or of those which may have damaged the heart should be adopted. If this is observed, no doubt a number of unnecessary operations will be undertaken but, on the other hand, no patient will be allowed to die of unrelieved or overlooked pericardial tamponade. Apart from stab wounds over the heart, skin wounds at a distance may be the entry wound of a weapon which has caused cardiac damage and epigastric and subcostal stabs are particularly sinister. All stab wounds of the chest and upper abdomen should be viewed with suspicion and, if cardiac injury is likely, exploration is advised (Hill, 1900; Beall et al., 1961).

Site of Exploration

Stab wounds on either side of the chest are best approached from the injured side, although from time to time a parasternal wound may be best exposed by way of median sternotomy. The patient admitted with a knife or other weapon embedded in his anterior chest wall presents a special problem. The weapon must not be disturbed lest fatal haemorrhage or tamponade occurs. The patient's survival is clearly dependent on the cardiac injury being sealed by the weapon, leaving adequate time for less desperate surgery. The patient is anaesthetized and draped for operation with the knife in place. The chest is opened anteriorly by an appropriate incision, the pericardium widely opened and only then is the weapon withdrawn. The bleeding is controlled by finger pressure and suturing undertaken.

FOREIGN BODIES IN THE HEART

The management of foreign bodies retained in the heart is controversial and considerable experience is available. Following early successful attempts at removal of bullets and shell fragments from the heart, further experience indicated that the mortality of expectant treatment was no greater than that of operative treatment, although in 1914 Sauerbruch advised removal of all foreign bodies from the heart and reported 105 cases with a mortality of 8 per cent. During World War II Harken (1946) and Swan et al. (1952) considered that recurrent pericardial effusion or infection were indications for surgical removal. Much of the sting has been removed from these arguments by the advent of cardiopulmonary by-pass for this allows a confident approach to the intracardiac foreign body. Bland and Beebe (1966) reported a 20-year follow-up of 40 patients with foreign bodies remaining in the heart following World War II. They noted that pericarditis was common and effusions occurred in 25 per cent, sometimes many years later. Removal was attempted in 8 of these patients. It was successful in 3 though the attempt was abandoned in 5. The problems created by intracardiac foreign bodies include those of migration and anxiety neurosis. These authors considered that once the foreign body is fixed in the myocardium migration is unlikely and erosion and infection were not seen during their 20-year follow-up.

It therefore seems wise to attempt the removal of foreign bodies from the heart as soon as possible after injury. However, if these are noted at a later date in the absence of symptoms their removal may not be necessary. Penetration of the heart by a missile may be complicated by damage to the septa or valves and murmurs should be assessed clinically and by cardiac catheterization.

PENETRATING INJURIES OF THE THORACIC AORTA

Although aortic rupture most commonly occurs in association with closed injuries, penetrating damage of the aorta caused by stab wounds, gunshot wounds or by shrapnel is becoming more frequent. Furthermore, because of improved methods of resuscitation and transit to traumatic centres, more of these patients are surviving emergency surgery. Whereas in patients with closed traumatic rupture of the aorta associated major injuries are extremely common, penetrating injuries of the aorta tend to be isolated and the dramatic nature of the injury and of the patient's condition makes early diagnosis likely.

The injury may be through and through or tangential, and when the aortic arch has been damaged transection of one or more great vessels from the aortic arch may occur. Injuries of the ascending aorta may be associated with pericardial tamponade and when the damage is caused by a low velocity missile this may remain within the vessel and subsequently migrate elsewhere in the arterial system.

Treatment

The site of exploration is of great importance and survival is usually associated with extremely early surgery. Cardiac arrest or sudden deterioration in the admitting room is an indication for immediate thoracotomy and in such circumstances simple control of the perforation by the thumb followed by suture of the wound may be life-saving.

Considering the nature of the injury, it is not surprising that preoperative evaluation by radiological means is unusual. Although it may be possible to obtain a chest radiograph, it is certainly unlikely that aortography will be available and subsequent surgery is therefore less tidy and definitive than that for closed aortic rupture. Nevertheless, in those centres where penetrating chest injuries are commonly seen, encouraging results of such treatment are emerging.

Reul and his colleagues (1974), from Houston, Texas, reported a series of such injuries and found penetrating wounds of the thoracic aorta to be equally distributed throughout the ascending, arch and descending aorta, and several patients with penetrating aortic trauma who had emergency room thoracotomy survived. Two of these had tangential wounds of the ascending aorta, with consequent pericardial tamponade in one, and both survived emergency surgery. Two had perforation of the ascending aorta and both had successful repair without the use of cardiopulmonary by-pass. Two further patients had perforating wounds of the ascending aorta and 1 survived. The seventh had penetration of the thoracic aorta with subsequent bullet embolus of the left ventricle and perforation of the pulmonary artery and right ventricle, and he survived after resuscitation and using left atriofemoral by-pass to facilitate repair. Five further patients had penetrating wounds of the descending thoracic aorta, of whom 3 survived. One of these had penetration of the thoracic aorta with distal bullet embolus to the profunda femoris artery and was treated successfully by aortic repair and embolectomy. A further group of 5 patients had aortic arch wounds and 3 of these were long term survivors following repair of the injury using cardiopulmonary by-pass.

The commonest cause of death in this series was, of course, failure to control haemorrhage. Nevertheless, the fact that such patients arrived in hospital alive suggests that the aortic wound may in many cases be amenable to life-saving repair. The principles of treatment of these patients should embrace immediate thoracotomy, control of the aortic wound and its suture with or without by-pass support. Other than in very specialized centres it is unlikely that by-pass support will be immediately available, and it therefore falls to the surgeon to do his best in the circumstances. Considering these limitations, it is surprising that many of these patients do in fact survive surgical treatment of such injuries. The majority are young and healthy which may protect them from the otherwise deleterious effects of temporary aortic cross clamping. Crawford and Rubio (1973) demonstrated the safety of aortic occlusion distal to the left subclavian artery in the resection of arteriosclerotic aneurysms of the thoracic aorta. Satisfactory protection of the spinal cord and distal vascular bed was obtained without heparinization, utilization of intravascular shunts or cardiopulmonary by-pass assistance and, although it is undoubtedly advisable to use by-pass support should it be available, it seems possible that it may not always be necessary, particularly in extreme emergencies (Billy et al., 1971).

Chapter 16

Penetrating wounds of the chest

Since penetrating wounds of the chest may cause cardiac, pulmonary and chest wall damage, it is convenient to consider some aspects of these injuries together, although some features may be discussed in more detail in other chapters.

These wounds are important for several problems may coexist:

1. Damage to intrathoracic structures.
2. Damage to abdominal organs.
3. Sucking pneumothorax.

Although knives, icepicks or low velocity bullets may cause limited damage often amenable to surgical treatment, the massive disruption caused by high velocity bullets, shotguns and battle injuries poses special and serious problems.

DAMAGE TO LUNGS, HEART OR MEDIASTINAL STRUCTURES

Pneumothorax or haemothorax is common and wounds of entry and exit are noted. The site and direction of these wounds may indicate possible cardiac involvement. The commonest of these wounds is fortunately the most innocuous, the isolated stab wound of the chest penetrated from behind or laterally which produces haemopneumothorax, and in these cases a conservative approach is advised in the first instance. Intercostal catheter drainage will remove air and blood and will be followed by full expansion of the lung. Usually the bleeding ceases and the air leak will close after a day or so, although continuous severe bleeding and air leak may require thoracotomy. Suspicion of cardiac injury requires careful monitoring of the patient's central venous pressure supported by frequent chest examinations and radiography. Deterioration in the patient's condition which could be explained by a cardiac injury is an indication for pericardiocentesis or for exploratory thoracotomy. Gunshot wounds usually require exploration whether or not the bullet remains in the chest. The rare exception to this rule is the patient with an entry and exit wound in the chest, well away from the heart whose haemopneumothorax responds rapidly and favourably to intercostal catheter drainage and does not reaccumulate.

PENETRATING DAMAGE TO THE DIAPHRAGM AND ABDOMINAL ORGANS

During full expiration the domes of the diaphragm may rise higher than the nipple lines and consequently the liver, spleen, stomach and parts of the colon may readily be damaged by an apparently uncomplicated stab wound of the chest. Any such wound below the nipple line anteriorly, laterally or posteriorly should be suspected of concomitant abdominal visceral damage and exploration advised (*Fig*. 45).

CASE REPORT

A 35-year-old man was admitted to the accident room with a stab wound 1·5 cm in size in the 7th intercostal space in the midaxillary line on the left side. Chest and abdominal examinations were normal and chest X-ray showed no evidence of air or fluid in the chest. The patient was observed for 4 hours and the wound sutured by a recently qualified doctor. The patient insisted on discharging himself but was fortunately persuaded not to do so. The patient was seen several hours later by a more experienced surgeon and although a further chest radiograph was reported as normal and there were no unusual symptoms, exploration was advised. The left chest was explored anteriorly with the incision crossing obliquely into the upper abdomen. It was found that the lower lobe of the left lung had been penetrated by the knife which had traversed the diaphragm, spleen and splenic flexure of the colon with considerable local soiling. Following attention to these injuries and after splenectomy the patient made an uninterrupted recovery.

SUCKING OR OPEN PNEUMOTHORAX (*Fig*. 46)

This is an urgent and life-threatening injury. Small perforations of the chest wall may produce a valve-like entry into the pleural cavity enabling air to be sucked into the pleura during inspiration and the valve occludes the perforation during expiration. A tension pneumothorax soon develops which endangers the patient, and subcutaneous emphysema may develop. Larger, more disruptive wounds of the

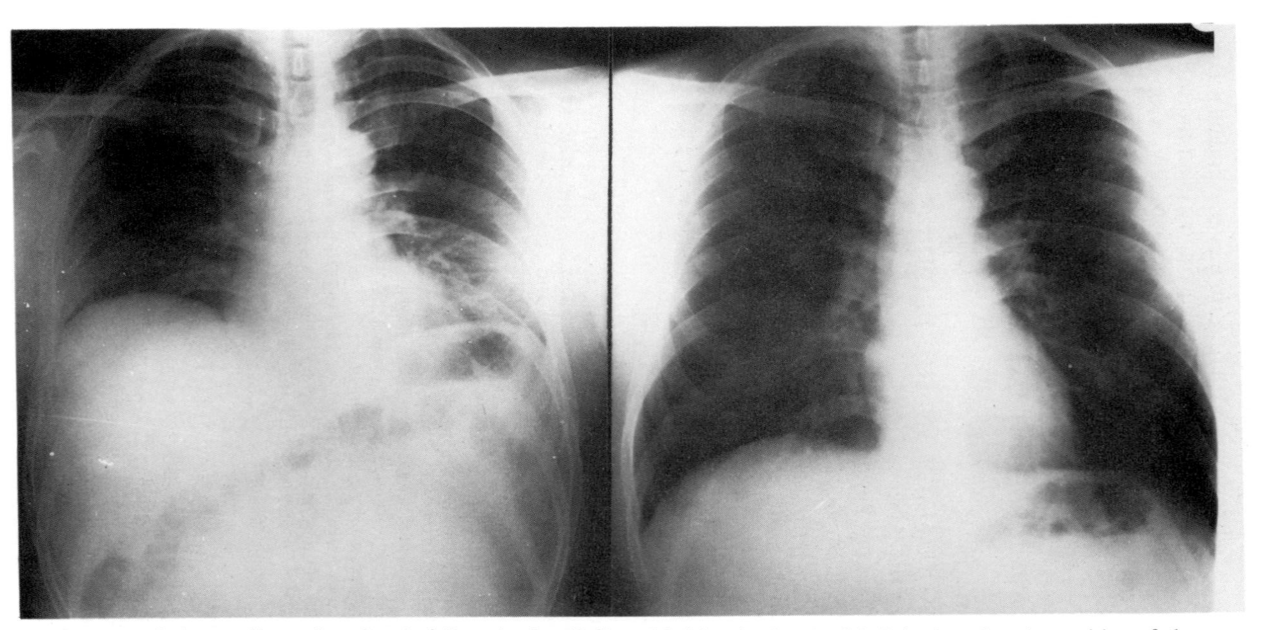

Fig. 45. Normal chest radiographs taken in full expiration (*left*) and full inspiration (*right*). It is clear that the position of the upper abdominal viscera varies considerably depending on the phase of respiration and that a penetrating wound in this area may produce an intrathoracic injury, an intra-abdominal injury or both of these

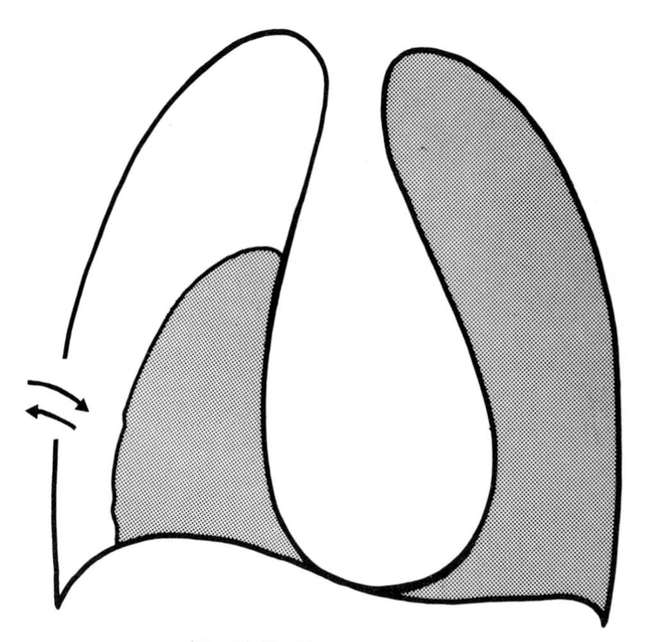

Fig. 46. Sucking pneumothorax.

chest wall may be caused by shotgun blast, shell injuries or penetration by wooden or metal fencing posts. Clothing and pieces of chest wall may be driven into the lung and be associated with loss of chest wall. Adequate ventilation is impossible.

Treatment

These patients are in a desperate condition and air is heard to suck in and out of the chest. The wound must be sealed with a dressing held firmly in place by adhesive strapping and an intercostal catheter introduced via a separate small stab incision. If the chest wound is large, operative débridement is necessary when dead tissue and loose bone are removed, the ribs and sternum wired and the defect closed. Should skin loss prevent direct closure, rotation of skin flaps from the abdominal wall or flank may be required.

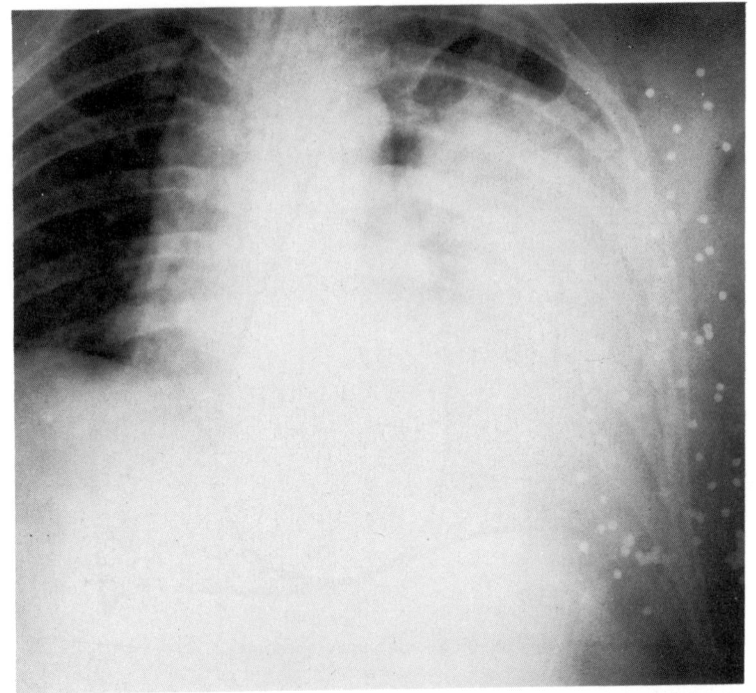

Fig. 47. Shotgun wound of chest. Although several ribs were shattered by the blast and the left lung was almost solid with oedema, there was no penetration of the chest by shot.

GUNSHOT AND SHRAPNEL WOUNDS OF THE CHEST
(*Figs.* 47 and 48)

These are particularly dangerous, for bullets, shrapnel, pellets and blast may have caused damage well away from entry or exit wounds. The shock wave will cause extensive contusion of the lung, even in the absence of penetration of that organ, and for this reason, tangential wounds of the chest wall by shotgun blast can cause fatal pulmonary oedema and contusion.

Failed attempts at suicide by shotgun injury are associated with disruption of the chest wall, lower lobe of the lung, diaphragm and upper abdominal organs on the left side. These wounds are compatible with survival, for major vessels and the heart are clearly unaffected. Nevertheless, the immediate problem of sucking pneumothorax must be urgently treated by the application of a large dressing to seal the wound. Operative débridement often requires lobectomy, splenectomy and, in the presence of large bowel injury, colostomy.

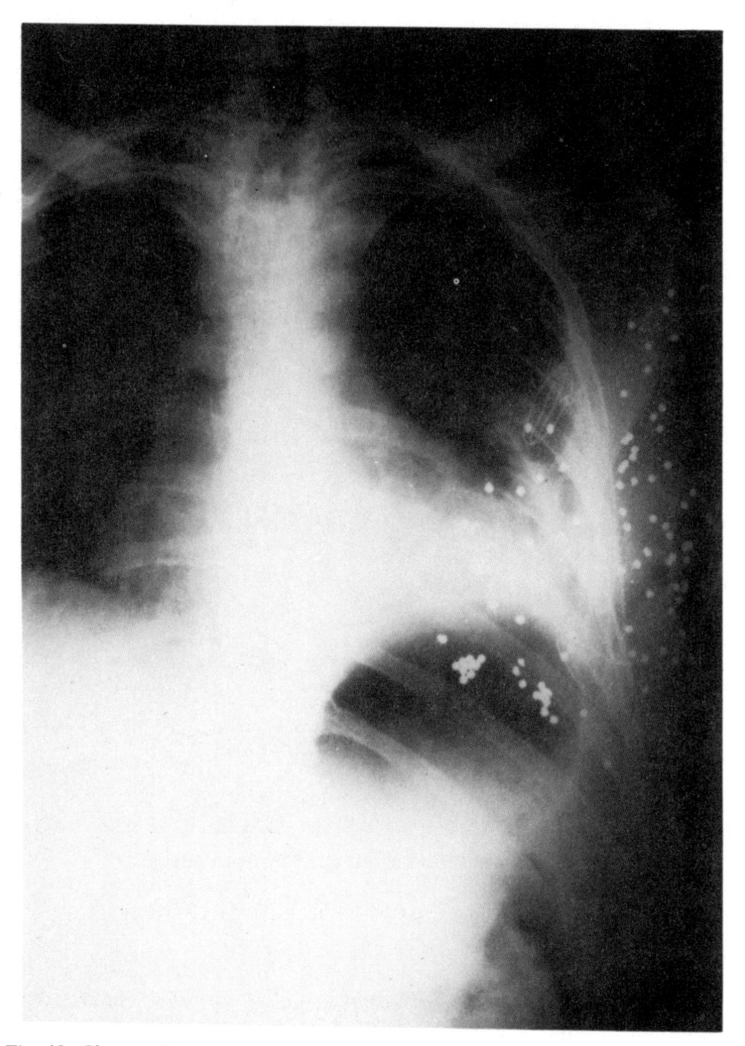

Fig. 48. Chest radiograph of patient in *Fig*. 47 following 1 week of intermittent positive pressure ventilation, which demonstrates almost complete clearing of the pulmonary contusion.

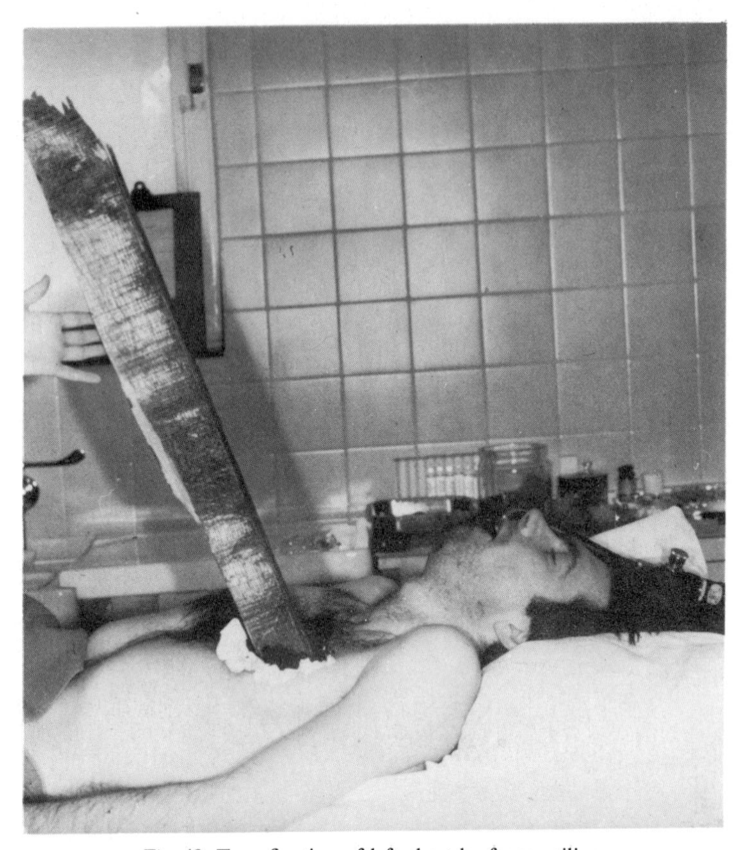

Fig. 49. Transfixation of left chest by fence railing.

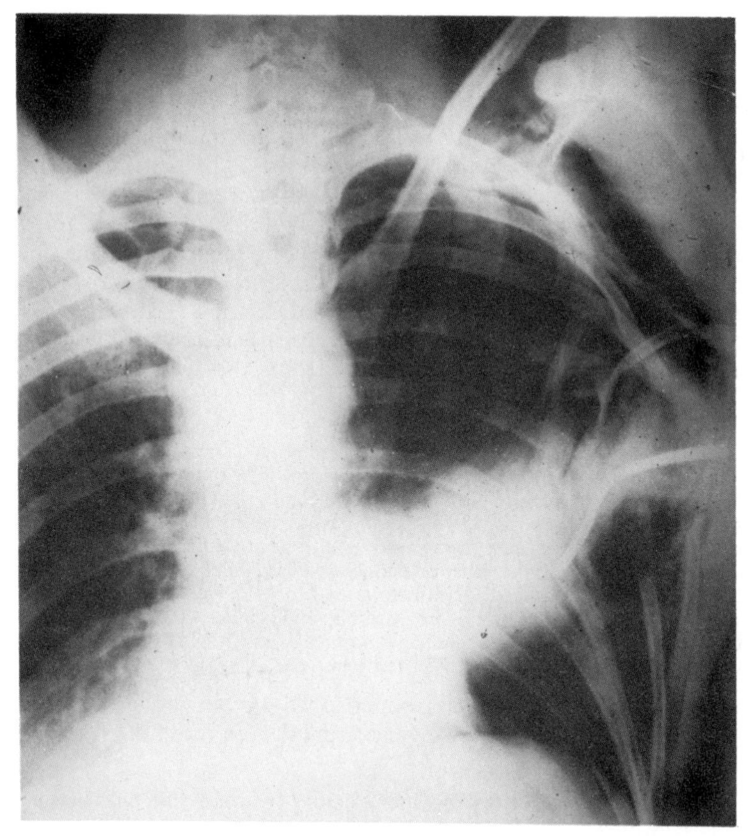

Fig. 50. Chest radiograph of patient in *Fig*. 49. Disruption of the chest wall is seen to be the main injury. The patient recovered following débridement and a period of intermittent positive pressure ventilation.

The problem of diaphragmatic and chest wall reconstruction may be extremely difficult. The associated major lung contusions usually respond well to positive pressure ventilation.

TRANSFIXATION INJURIES OF THE CHEST

Transfixation of the chest by metal or wooden railings may be associated with high speed motor accidents, and from time to time such patients are admitted to hospital with the railing still in place. Usually the railing has penetrated subcutaneously or deep to the chest wall muscles, but other than breaking adjacent ribs has not penetrated the thoracic cavity. Such injuries respond to simple débridement and treatment of associated injuries. Several cases of more severe transfixation have been reported and the case described by Marable and Maloney in 1963 is startling.

CASE REPORT

A 24 × 2 × 4 in fence rail penetrated the chest of an 18-year-old boy who had been involved in a high speed sports car accident. The railing entered his chest at the right of the sternum detaching the 2nd to 6th right costal cartilages from the sternum and fracturing the sternum, passing across the front of the heart and pericardium displacing them posteriorly, disrupting the upper lobe of the left lung and avulsing the superior pulmonary vein. After traversing the upper lobe the rail had fractured the 4th rib lateral to its angle, and penetrated the chest posteriorly between the left scapula and spine. Appropriate surgical treatment was carried out, including resection of much of the left upper lobe and the patient made an uneventful recovery. (*Figs*. 49 and 50.)

The fact that this case responded to heroic modern surgical treatment makes the following case report even more interesting.

CASE REPORT

In 1841 Earle reported the case of Thomas Tipple. Thomas Tipple, on the evening of 13 June, 1812, began to unharness a horse, but being inexperienced he started by taking off the bridle. When this had been removed the horse sprang forwards and the end of one of the shafts of the gig struck Tipple upon the left breast, piercing the chest wall, traversed a portion of the thorax and came out upon the right side and penetrated the wall of the house. He was found standing on tiptoe with both arms extended. Although completely impaled he was able to put his hands on the end of the shaft and help to draw himself off. He was seen by William Maiden and Sir William Blizzard in consultation, who prognosticated a fatal termination before morning. Despite these predictions, however, Tipple survived. His treatment over the next 10 days consisted of venesection of a total of 132 ounces of blood, the application of blisters to the wound and the administration of enemas.

These case reports remind us that patients have in the past from time to time survived dreadful injuries without surgical treatment and that the prognosis is usually dependent on the degree of damage to vital structures.

Chapter 17

Closed injuries of the thoracic aorta and great vessels

It is almost unbelievable that anyone survives closed traumatic rupture of the aorta, but an appreciable number of such patients do reach hospital alive.

A review of 296 fatal cases of injury of the aorta extracted from the files of the U.S. Armed Forces Institute of Pathology showed that 38 (13 per cent) survived initially (Parmley, Mattingly and Manion, 1958). Survival is dependent on the formation of an acute false aneurysm contained by the adventitial layer and mediastinal structures. This aneurysm may rupture within minutes, hours or days. In patients who initially survive without evidence of aortic injury an unsuspected aortic aneurysm may rupture months or years later. Still others may develop post-traumatic aneurysm which may remain silent until detected by routine chest radiography.

INCIDENCE

The incidence of traumatic rupture of the aorta has markedly increased with the development of rapid travel, and post-traumatic aneurysm is now the commonest thoracic aortic aneurysm in the young. Seventy-two acute aortic ruptures were found among 7000 consecutive autopsies performed in Manhatten between the years 1936 and 1942, and 70 per cent of these were the result of motor vehicle accidents (Strassman, 1947). In a series of 250 fatal road accidents 14 fatal aortic ruptures were found, some of which had finally ruptured hours or days after the injury and might have been amenable to surgery (Sevitt, 1968).

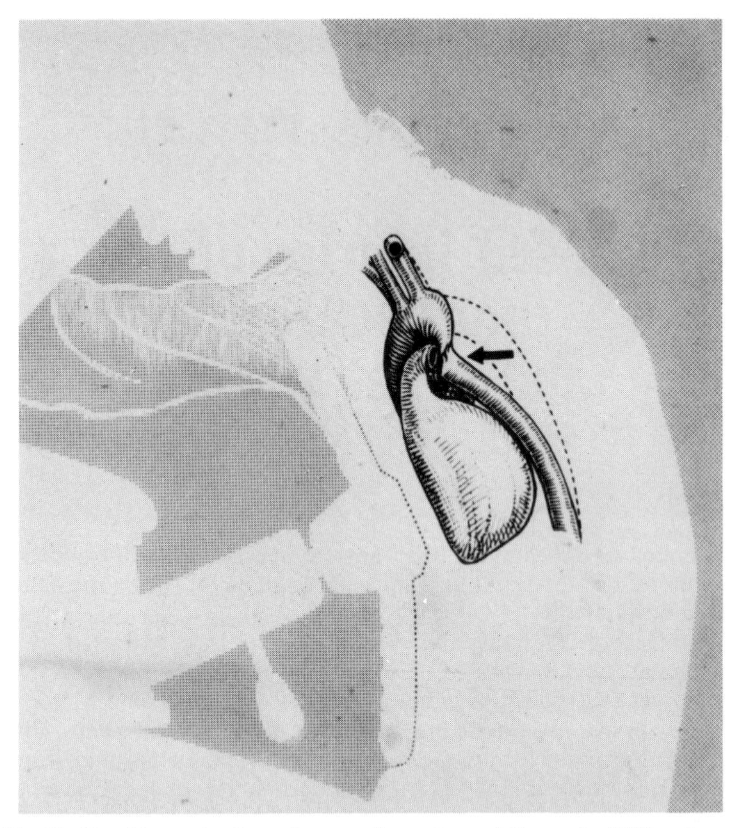

Fig. 51. Possible mechanism of traumatic rupture of the aorta. With extreme deceleration the lower thoracic aorta continues to whiplash forwards with consequent tearing of the aorta at the ligamentum arteriosum.

In Bristol 37 such patients out of a population of 600 000 came to either surgery or autopsy in a 6-year period. Most patients were males and the average age was in the late twenties (Keen, 1972).

AETIOLOGY AND SITE

Traumatic rupture of the aorta follows either rapid deceleration or direct chest injury. Most of the patients are victims of motor car accidents, air crashes or falls from a height. Among more unusual injuries reported are a kick by a calf (Spencer et al., 1961) and sudden burial by an earth fall. Traumatic rupture of the aorta was discovered at autopsy in 8 out of 28 victims of an air crash (Teare,

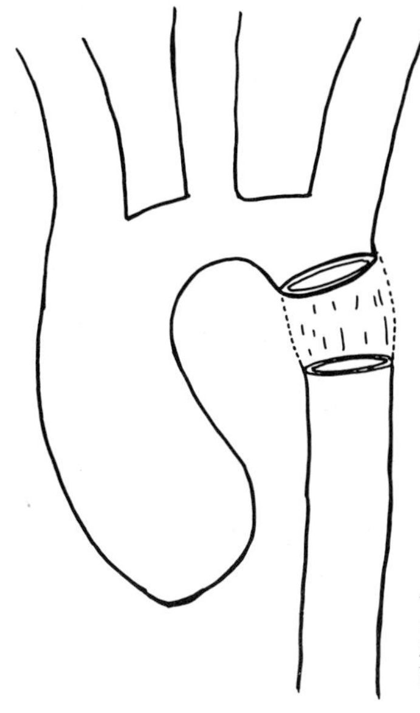

Fig. 52. Traumatic rupture of the aorta. Although there is wide separation of the media, the false aneurysm is contained by the adventitia.

1951), and in the large American series of 296 fatal cases 70 per cent followed car accidents, 15 per cent air crashes, and the remainder had either crushing injuries or direct trauma (Parmley, Mattingly and Manion, 1958).

The mechanism of aortic rupture with deceleration may be related to different deceleration rates between fixed and more mobile parts. Thus in violent deceleration the relatively free descending thoracic aorta is snapped forwards at a different rate from the fixed portions of the aorta, and such unequal deceleration subjects the aorta to stretch, torsion and shearing stress, with rupture at these fixed points (*Fig*. 51). An alternative suggestion is the avulsion of heart and aortic arch from the aorta at the ligamentum which occurs as the heart is projected forwards and upwards in violent deceleration. Thus it is that the aorta is most frequently damaged at its isthmus, i.e. the segment between the left subclavian artery and the ligamentum arteriosum (*Fig*. 52).

Injuries of the ascending aorta and aortic vessels are more likely to follow direct trauma than deceleration, and in injuries of these vessels it is common to find fractures and fracture dislocations in the region of the anterior chest wall overlying these vessels. Falls on to the feet may rupture the ascending aorta by avulsion of the junction of the fixed aortic arch and the mobile heart. Such tears are often associated with aortic valvular injury. In Parmley's series of 296 cases 80 per cent of ruptures occurred at the isthmus or just below (Parmley, Mattingly and Manion, 1958), and in my own experience of 20 patients 17 (85 per cent) had aortic ruptures at or below the isthmus and the remainder ruptures of either the innominate or subclavian vessels (Keen, 1972).

PATHOLOGY AND PROGRESS

Traumatic rupture of the aorta has the appearance of an incised wound extending transversely or spirally, partially or completely, around the vessel, involving part or all of the vessel thickness (*Fig.* 53). There is no evidence to suggest that existing disease such as medial necrosis, atheroma or syphilitic aortitis predisposes to traumatic rupture of the aorta, and the histological appearance of the aorta in these patients (most of whom are young) is usually normal. In 1728 Nicholls experimentally overdistended the pulmonary artery at autopsy and produced bursting of the internal coats, with the formation of an aneurysmal outpouching of the external coats, a similar injury to that seen in traumatic rupture of the aorta. It has been shown that a pressure of between 1000 and 3000 mmHg is required to rupture the aorta (Oppenheim, 1918). Should complete rupture of all layers take place immediate exsanguination is likely, although some have survived surgery after this injury.

In those who reach hospital alive there is commonly rupture of the intima and media, the ends of which may be retracted several centimetres apart and continuity is retained by a sheath of intact adventitia (*Fig.* 54). This sheath may contain the aortic pressure, although rupture usually follows in due course. If the aorta is examined shortly after injury and during thoracotomy for another injury, such as ruptured diaphragm, it may appear normal, and several cases have been recorded in which this injury was overlooked at exploratory thoracotomy. One such patient was found to have an apparently normal aorta at operation, despite a clinical diagnosis of ruptured aorta, and aortotomy was therefore not carried out. However, he developed an obvious aneurysm clearly seen on chest radiographs 3 weeks later and at further operation the aortic wall was found to be completely transected just below the left subclavian artery, with a 6-cm separation of the aortic ends leading into the aneurysmal sac (Eiseman and Rainer, 1958). One of my own patients died

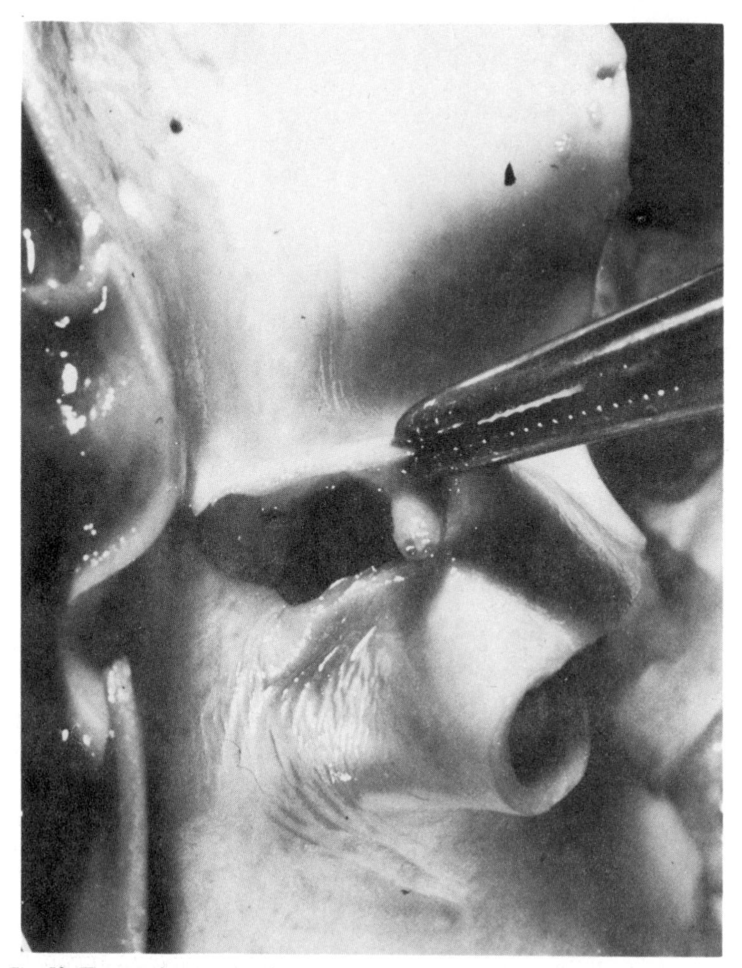

Fig. 53. Traumatic rupture of aorta at the level of the ligamentum. This patient died suddenly 4 hours after leaping from a high staircase following the use of a hallucinatory drug.

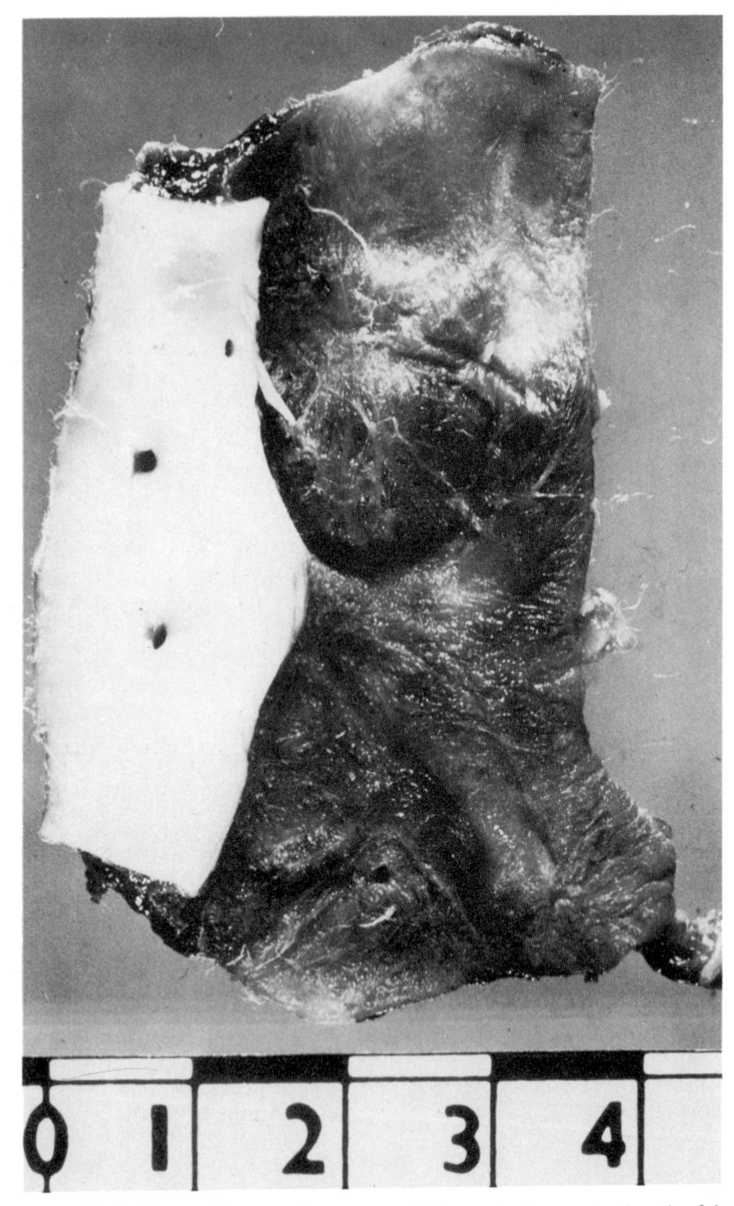

Fig. 54. Excised area of traumatic rupture of the aorta demonstrating the false aneurysm to be of adventitia only.

unexpectedly of aortic rupture 9 days after thoracotomy for ruptured diaphragm, when the aorta appeared normal.

CASE REPORT

A man, aged 28, who had been involved in a motor accident was admitted to hospital in 1965. He was concussed and had fractures of the ribs, pelvis and left femur. Radiologically there was rupture of the left diaphragm with herniation of abdominal contents into the thorax (*Fig.* 55). Operation was undertaken several hours later. The left pleural cavity contained stomach, omentum, transverse colon and spleen. The abdominal viscera were replaced and the diaphragm, which had a large radial tear, was repaired. No other abnormality was noted. A Steinmann pin was inserted into the left tibial tubercle for traction. Although apparently well, he had anuria after the operation and dialysis was required. Haemodialysis was undertaken twice, but on the 9th postoperative day he suddenly collapsed and died. At autopsy there was a 2-cm tear of the posterior aspect of aorta at the ligamentum arteriosum. Blood had been contained within a small sac of adventitia which had ruptured. Review of chest radiographs taken on admission and on the day before death showed the mediastinal shadow to be widened and, had this sign been noted, the diagnosis might have been suspected earlier, with the possibility of successful treatment (*Fig.* 56).

In some cases the acute traumatic aneurysm may enlarge to form a false chronic aneurysm, its lining of thickened adventitia stretching to the point of rupture months or years later or progressing to calcification of the wall and a so-called 'stable' state.

CASE REPORT

A 25-year-old man presented at Westminster Hospital in 1956, having been referred from the Mass Miniature Radiography Centre. He had no symptoms. Radiographs showed a mass 6 cm in diameter in the posterior mediastinum on the left side which was considered to be a mediastinal cyst. Exploratory thoracotomy showed this to be an aneurysm of the thoracic aorta just below the origin of the left subclavian artery and this was not disturbed. The patient subsequently said that 5 years earlier he had been involved in an accident in an international cycle race and had woken up in hospital 2 days later with a headache and a sore chest. Apparently no chest radiograph had been taken. The patient was seen 4 years after exploration, when radiography showed the aneurysm to be unchanged in size, although calcification of its wall was now noted. Surgery was refused. The patient was well 20 years after his injury, and the radiograph was unchanged (*Fig.* 57).

The dangers of rupture, compression, erosion and infection are always present. One of my patients suffered progressive compression of the left main bronchus with apparent imminent rupture into this structure.

CASE REPORT

A 30-year-old man was referred in 1969 with traumatic aneurysm of the aorta. He had been knocked down by a car 3 years earlier when laparotomy was

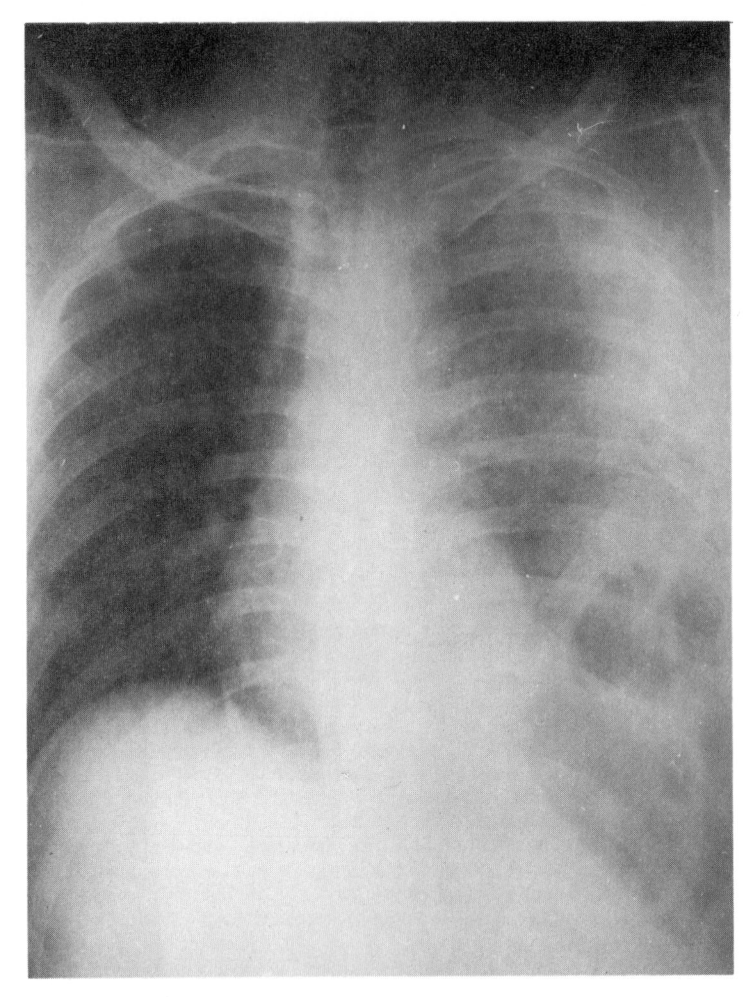

Fig. 55. Traumatic rupture of aorta and traumatic rupture of left diaphragm following chest injury. Unfortunately, the latter injury only was diagnosed and the patient died suddenly 9 days later.

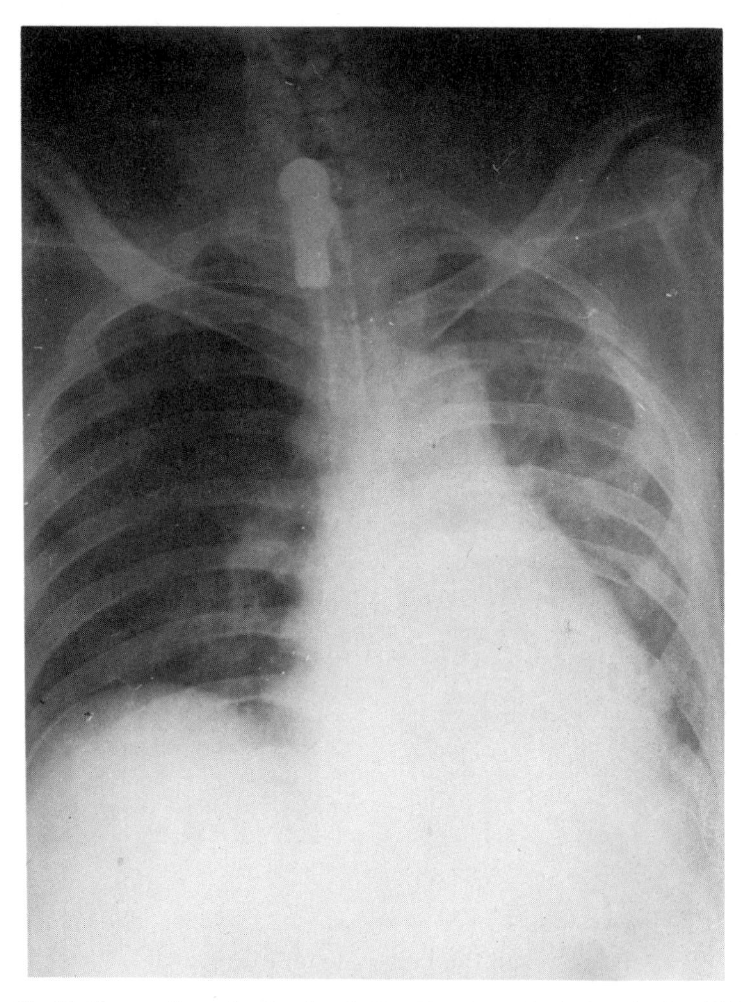

Fig. 56. Chest radiograph of patient in *Fig*. 55, taken 1 day before death, which clearly shows a mediastinal haematoma. This was not noted.

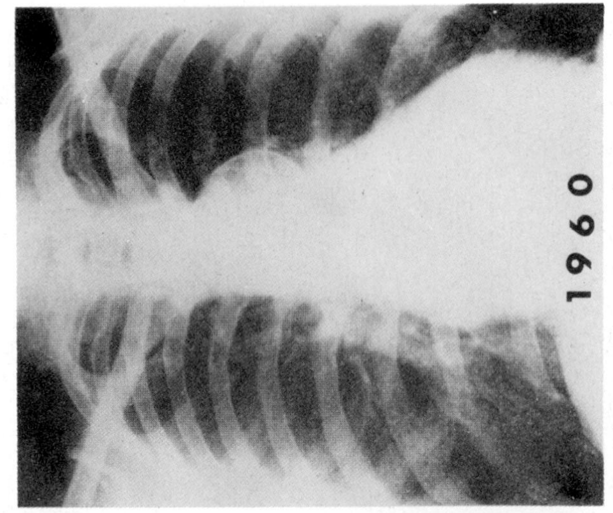

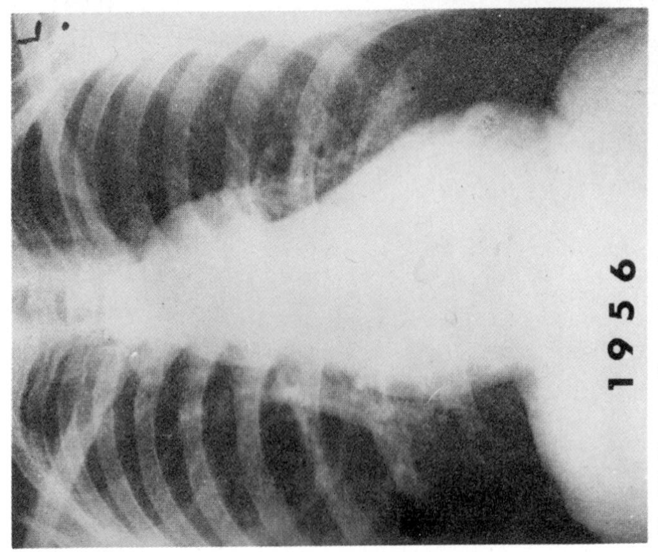

Fig. 57. Chest radiographs of patient with traumatic aneurysm of the descending thoracic aorta. In the 4-year interval that elapsed between the two radiographs calcification of the wall has occurred.

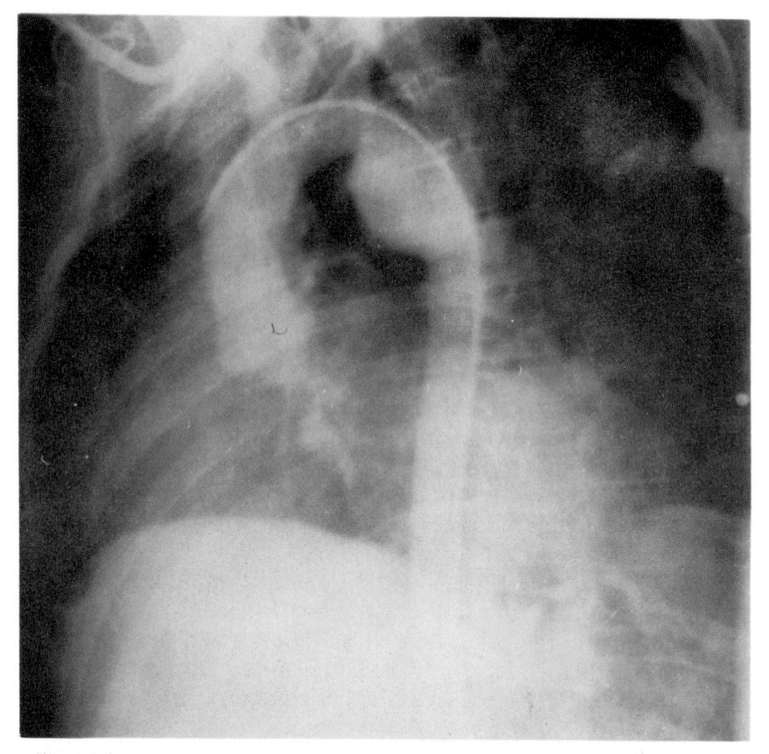

Fig. 58. Traumatic aneurysm of the aorta causing left bronchial compression.

undertaken on account of suspected ruptured spleen and diaphragm. At the time of the present admission he had no symptoms other than chronic cough. Chest X-ray showed a saccular aneurysm distal to the left subclavian artery which was confirmed at aortography (*Fig.* 58). Bronchoscopy was undertaken because of chronic cough and the left main bronchus was found to be reduced to a narrow anteroposterior slit, the lateral wall of which pulsated in a most alarming fashion. Resection of the aneurysm was advised. It was the size of half an egg and was compressing and adherent to the left main bronchus, the lateral wall of which was reduced to tissue-paper thickness. Using left atriofemoral by-pass the aneurysm was resected and replaced with a woven Dacron graft, after which the patient made an uninterrupted recovery. It seems likely that if undisturbed this aneurysm would have ruptured into the left main bronchus.

A soldier developed acute superior vena caval obstruction 48 days after chest injury and died of a ruptured ascending aortic aneurysm some days later (Parmley, Mattingly and Manion, 1958). An 18-year-old girl died of septicaemia 6 months after chest injury and was found at autopsy to have a traumatic aneurysm of the ascending thoracic aorta which was infected (Stryker, 1948). Several experienced authors describe patients who harboured apparently safe post-traumatic aneurysms of the aorta which ultimately ruptured years after the original injury (DeBakey, 1968; Cooley, 1969). A patient presented with chronic traumatic aneurysm of the aorta 17 years after an air crash, after which he seemed unharmed. Chest radiography showed the aneurysm to be enlarging and this was associated with pain in the chest and back. Resection of the aneurysm was advised, but it ruptured 2 days before the planned operation (Slaney et al., 1966). A patient ruptured his traumatic aneurysm while playing cards 6 years after a motor car injury but fortunately survived emergency surgery (Sondergaard, 1970). In another patient a traumatic aortic aneurysm did not change in size radiologically for 14 years but then rapidly enlarged over a 3-year period to massive proportions (Spencer et al., 1961). There were 2 patients in the author's own series with ruptured post-traumatic aneurysms, 2 years after injury in one, who died, and 8 years after injury in the other, who survived emergency surgery.

Against this generally gloomy prognostic background others paint a rosy picture. One author described 5 patients with traumatic aneurysm of the thoracic aorta whose injuries had been sustained 2–27 years earlier, and the only patient who died did so after surgery and the remainder did well. On the basis of this small series and in the context of surgical practice at that time (1957) conservatism was advised (Steinberg, 1957). However, there is no doubt that post-traumatic aortic aneurysms should be resected in most instances, having regard to the age and general condition of the patient.

Most of these patients have other major injuries, and indeed in some fatal cases it is difficult to decide which of many injuries was responsible for death. On the other hand, patients who have sustained rupture of the aorta may have no other apparent injury. A 19-year-old boy who walked into a hospital casualty department shortly after a motor cycle accident, with his only apparent injury being a scalp laceration, developed rapidly progressive paraplegia 2 hours later and died of ruptured aorta shortly afterwards (Slaney et al., 1966). In the author's own experience of 20 such patients most had associated major injuries, including ruptured diaphragm in 5, ruptured spleen in 6, and major fractures in the majority. All had head injuries ranging in severity from mild concussion to fatal brain damage. It is not surprising that aortic damage was often initially overlooked. One series of 15 patients with traumatic rupture of the aorta has been reported in which aortic rupture went unrecognized until autopsy in 7 of the 11 who died. Furthermore, in these cases the diagnosis had never been entertained (Demeules et al., 1971).

CLINICAL DIAGNOSIS

The keystone of diagnosis is a high index of suspicion and the possibility should always be considered in cases of high speed trauma or after crushing injury to the chest. In these patients chest radiography is essential. Chest pain is not diagnostic but later onset of pain radiating to the back may be a feature and is considered to be caused by further dissection and stripping of the sensitive aortic layers. Several authors have noted the onset of upper limb hypertension associated with a systolic murmur, attributed to reflex sympathetic aortic spasm or aortic obstruction (Rice and Wittstruck, 1951; Spencer et al., 1961).

Abnormalities of the peripheral pulses are sometimes noted, and in patients with traumatic rupture of the subclavian artery arm pulses are absent although carotid arterial pulses are present and equal. Ischaemic damage to the spinal cord with paraplegia may occur in the event of total interruption of aortic blood flow or avulsion of intercostal vessels (Spencer et al., 1961; Hughes, 1964; Slaney et al., 1966).

RADIOLOGY

With traumatic rupture of the aorta there is usually radiological widening of the mediastinum. However, in the presence of pneumothorax, haemothorax, ruptured diaphragm or surgical emphysema mediastinal widening may not be so apparent, and the lack of good quality radiographs associated with emergency radiography adds to the difficulties. The significance of deviation of the intrathoracic trachea to the right in mediastinal haematoma of aortic origin has been stressed (Sandor, 1967). The importance of careful scrutiny of the chest radiograph cannot be over-emphasized and from a review of the literature and of the author's own cases it is apparent that numerous patients have died because the presence and significance of mediastinal widening were not appreciated.

CASE REPORT

A 40-year-old man who had crashed his car was admitted to hospital. On examination he was found to have surgical emphysema of the right chest and a fractured right femur. While under anaesthesia for insertion of a Steinmann's pin and suture of a lacerated scalp he had cardiac arrest, from which he was resuscitated by external cardiac massage. Fifteen hours later his condition deteriorated and a further chest radiograph showed the left chest to be opaque (*Fig*. 59). Immediate thoracotomy was undertaken, but as the chest was opened it was clear that the aorta had ruptured completely, its ends being 10 cm apart

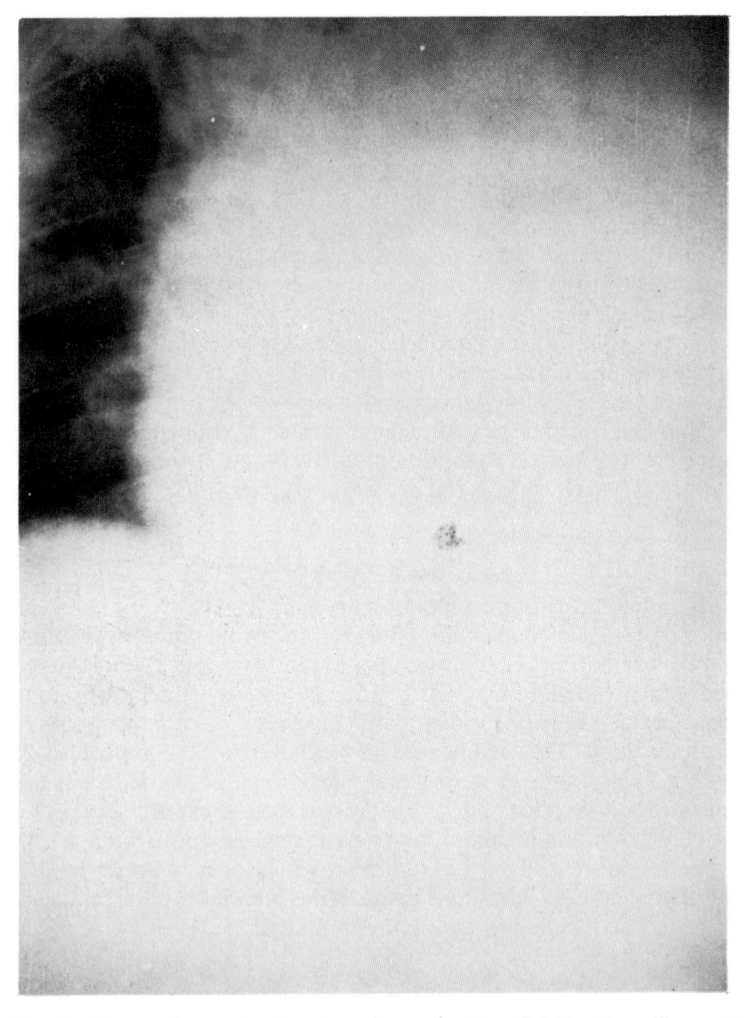

Fig. 59. Chest radiograph of patient shown in *Fig*. 60 following collapse 18 hours after injury. The chest radiograph demonstrates a large haemothorax and at emergency operation this was confirmed to be due to wide disruption of the thoracic aorta.

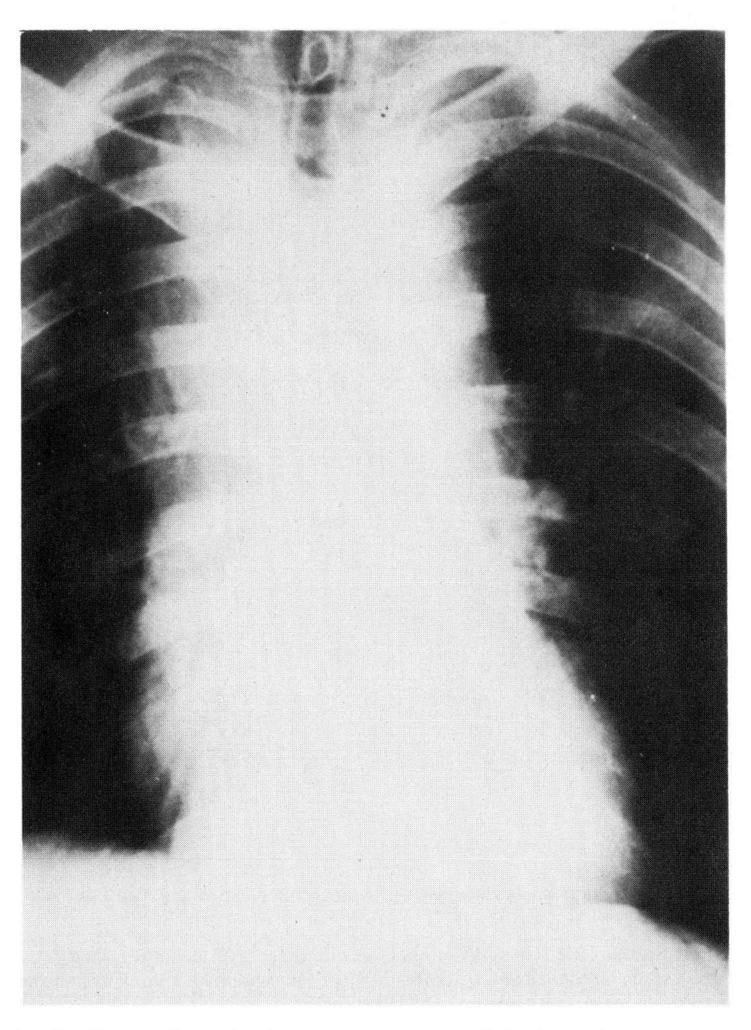

Fig. 60. Chest radiograph of patient taken 1 hour following serious motor car accident which demonstrated the presence of a large mediastinal haematoma. This radiograph was not examined until after the patient had collapsed and died 17 hours later.

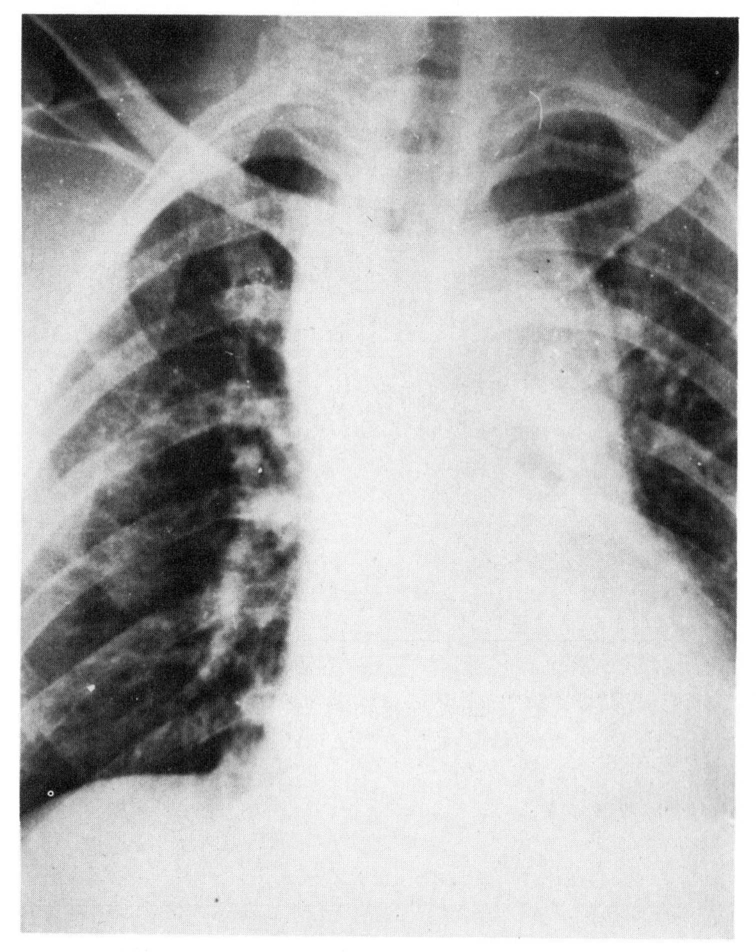

Fig. 61. Traumatic mediastinal haematoma following a 20-ft fall.

and he died almost at once, 18 hours after admission. Review of the chest radiograph, taken at the time of admission but not examined until later, showed clearly a widened mediastinum (*Fig.* 60).

Aortography is necessary both to confirm the presence and locate the site of aortic rupture; it will also help to avoid unnecessary surgery in patients with more benign causes of mediastinal bleeding (*Figs.* 61 and 62). Patients are encountered with mediastinal haematoma following injury in whom aortography is normal and in

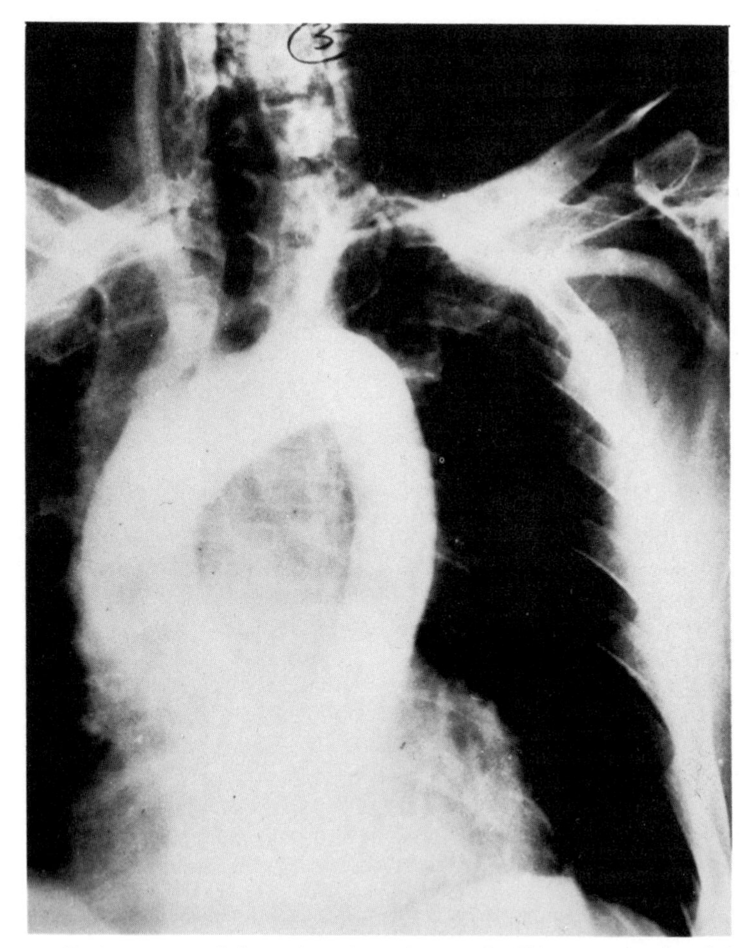

Fig. 62. Aortogram of the patient shown in *Fig*. 61. This was normal and the haematoma was considered a consequence of ruptured mediastinal veins. The patient made an uninterrupted recovery.

whom thoracotomy is unnecessary. Surgery without the benefit of aortographic confirmation is not advised, for when an operation has been performed without it, an aortic rupture has been missed altogether or a second rupture overlooked (Eiseman and Rainer, 1958; Passaro and Pace, 1959). Aortography is safe and reliable and should be carried out on all patients with traumatic mediastinal haematoma. It is best undertaken percutaneously via either the

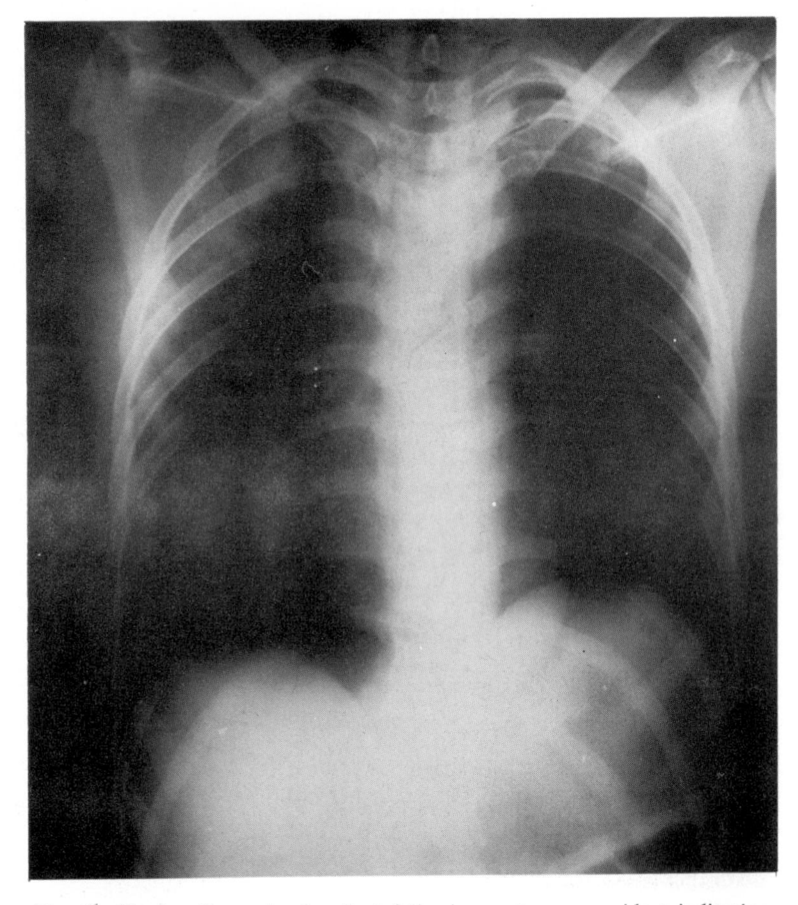

Fig. 63. Chest radiograph of patient following motor car accident indicating mediastinal haematoma.

femoral or the brachial artery. In the early days of aortography for this condition the transvenous route was used, and subsequently radiologists have employed the transventricular and trans-septal routes, although few radiologists would now choose transcardiac methods on account of their specialized nature. Most prefer trans-femoral aortography, and no case of perforation of the aneurysm by the catheter has been recorded. Femoral puncture has the added advantage that, if necessary, the descending thoracic and abdominal aorta can be investigated easily. With the mouth of the catheter

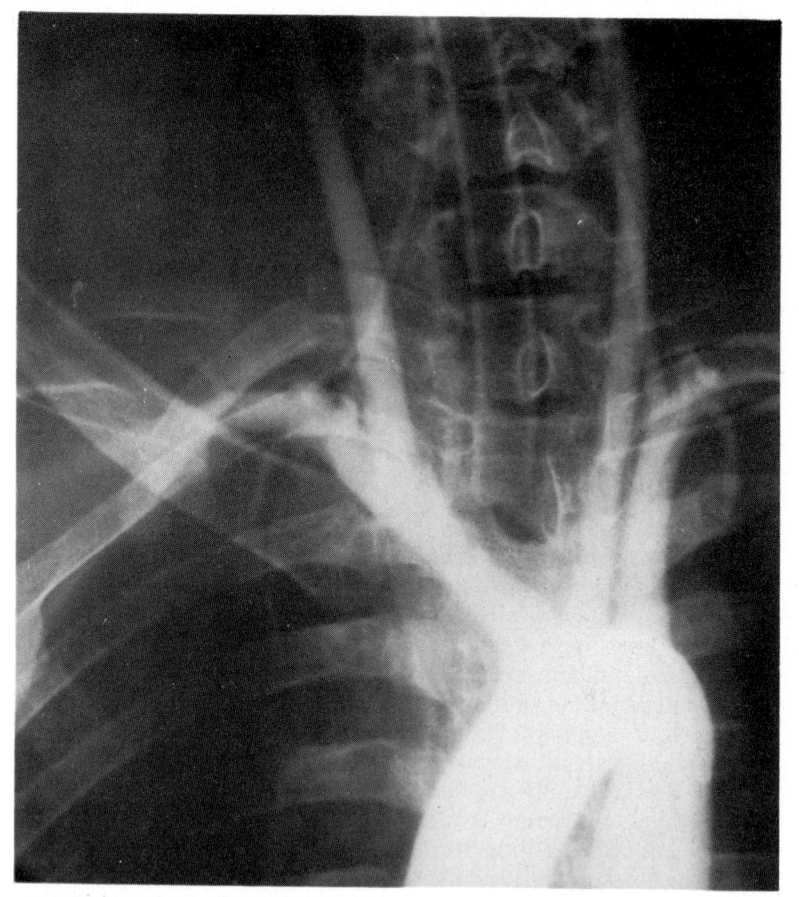

Fig. 64. Aortogram of patient shown in *Fig.* 63 demonstrating rupture of the distal innominate artery.

placed just above the aortic valve aortography will clearly demonstrate the whole of the thoracic aorta and its main branches (*Figs.* 63 and 64).

MANAGEMENT

Eighty-five per cent of patients with traumatic rupture of the aorta die before reaching hospital and of the 15 per cent who survive the majority will die of secondary haemorrhage within the next 10 days in the absence of treatment. A small number will survive and develop chronic aneurysms and many of these will suffer further complications from their aneurysms. For these reasons early repair should be attempted in most patients with acute traumatic rupture of the aorta, with the exception of those clearly dying of other injuries.

Similarly, most post-traumatic aortic aneurysms should be resected in view of the likelihood of rupture. It would, however, be difficult to make a case for resecting a symptomless post-traumatic aneurysm of the aorta in an elderly patient whose injury had been sustained many years earlier.

The operative approach and techniques used differ, depending on the site of the aneurysm. Those occurring beyond the left subclavian artery require a local form of by-pass, whereas lesions more proximal pose the problem of protection of the brain from ischaemic damage during surgery.

SURGERY OF INJURIES OF THE DESCENDING THORACIC AORTA

Operation is complicated by the need to cross-clamp the aorta high up and at the same time to prevent left ventricular strain and protect the kidneys, spinal cord and abdominal viscera from the effects of ischaemia. In experimental animals aortic cross-clamping at this level without by-pass results in a marked rise in left ventricular, left atrial and pulmonary artery pressure, and if aortic occlusion is maintained for longer than about 20 minutes at normal temperatures the risk of paraplegia is very real (Kahn, 1970; Taber, 1970).

In the first reported successful repair of traumatic rupture of the aorta (Passaro and Pace, 1959), the surgeon cross-clamped the aorta of a 30-year-old man without by-pass for a 17-minute period, during which he sutured a 3-mm tear at the isthmus. He noted that the heart became grossly distended and the electrocardiograph pattern bizarre, with conduction defects and T-wave inversion, and that the proximal blood pressure rose to 200 mmHg. Although the patient survived, this experience was sufficiently worrying to persuade the surgeon to recommend hypothermia on future occasions. Others consider that patients in whom restorative surgery is undertaken rapidly have no need of by-pass support (Crawford et al., 1970). However, this view takes no account of possible renal damage, especially in the elderly, and the risk of paraplegia is by no means illusory.

Paraplegia following surgery of the descending thoracic aorta may be due in part to the disease process itself, as with dissecting aneurysms, or to excessive sacrifice of intercostal vessels. The main branch to the anterior spinal artery supplying the spinal cord originates from the region of the lower thoracic and upper lumbar segmental vessels and interference in this area is liable to produce spinal cord ischaemia. In coarctation of the aorta collaterals will support the distal circulation during resection but in acute traumatic rupture or chronic aneurysms no such mechanism exists. Having regard to the dangers of cardiac dilatation and strain on the one hand and paraplegia on the other, such surgery without by-pass seems reckless. Various methods of countering these dangers have been described.

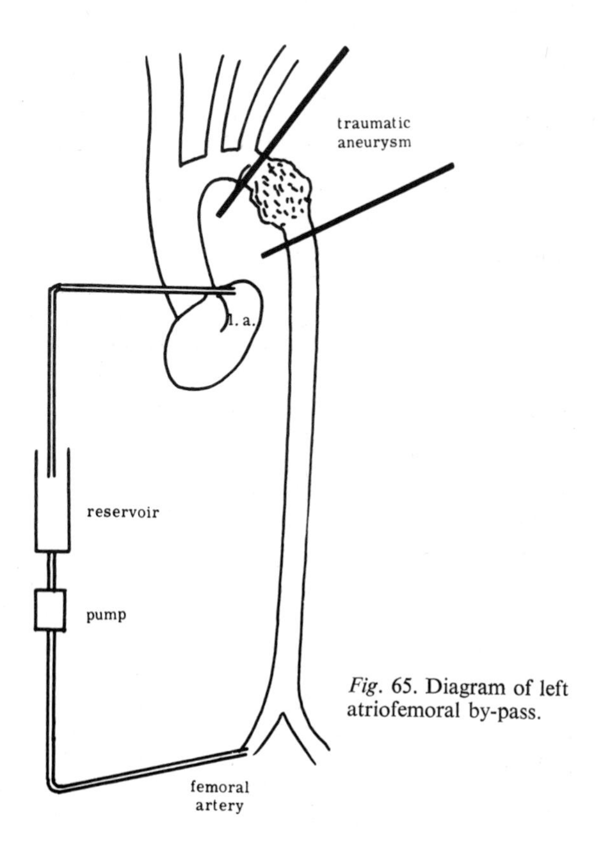

Fig. 65. Diagram of left atriofemoral by-pass.

LEFT ATRIOFEMORAL BY-PASS (Cooley et al., 1957; Gerbode et al., 1957) (*Fig*. 65; *see also Figs*. 66, 67 and 75).

This technique allows satisfactory operating conditions, preventing proximal hypertension and left ventricular strain during aortic cross-clamping and ensures adequate renal and spinal cord perfusion. Heparinization and its reversal by protamine pose no undue problems, unless there is intra-abdominal or intracerebral bleeding, when heparinization might aggravate this. The patient is positioned on the operating table in the right lateral position, i.e. with the left chest uppermost, with the pelvis rotated 45° backwards and the left hip joint fully extended. The chest is exposed for full thoracotomy and access is provided to the femoral vessels. The left femoral artery is first prepared for cannulation and the chest is opened widely through the 4th intercostal space. Alternatively, distal perfusion may be undertaken directly into the aorta below the occluding clamp. Before mobilization of the aorta the pericardium is opened posteriorly to the phrenic nerve and the left atrial appendage snared by a purse-string. These precautions allow for immediate left atriofemoral by-pass should haemorrhage occur during dissection of the acute aortic rupture. A large-bore cannula is introduced into the left atrium, whence blood is drained by gravity into an open reservoir or a disposable oxygenator and then returned via a roller pump to the femoral artery or distal thoracic aorta. Heparinization is required in a dose of 1 mg per kg body weight and is subsequently reversed with protamine in similar amounts. A distal flow rate of 40 ml per kg body weight per minute ensures decompression of the proximal aorta with adequate perfusion of the kidneys and spinal cord. During perfusion the radial arterial pressure should be maintained at 80 mmHg and urinary flow indicates adequacy of renal perfusion.

CASE REPORT

A 54-year-old man was admitted to hospital in 1967 after a car accident. His injuries included concussion and central dislocation of the right hip. Chest radiography showed the mediastinal shadow to be rather large. He had undergone transthoracic repair of hiatus hernia 10 years earlier and a follow-up radiograph taken 5 months before the accident was fortunately available. Comparison with the present radiograph showed obvious alteration in the size of the mediastinal shadow (*Fig*. 66). Aortography showed an almost complete circumferential tear of the aorta just below the subclavian artery (*Fig* 67). At thoracotomy with left atriofemoral by-pass the aortic haematoma was dissected and transection confirmed. It proved impossible to perform a satisfactory end-to-end anastomosis and the gap was therefore bridged with a 3-cm length of woven Dacron, after which the patient made an uneventful recovery.

MODERATE HYPOTHERMIA AT 30 °C

This has now been superseded by by-pass procedures, and was used when surface cooling had an important place in cardiac and vascular surgery. Although several successful cases of suture of ruptured aortas and resection of thoracic aneurysms have been reported, the

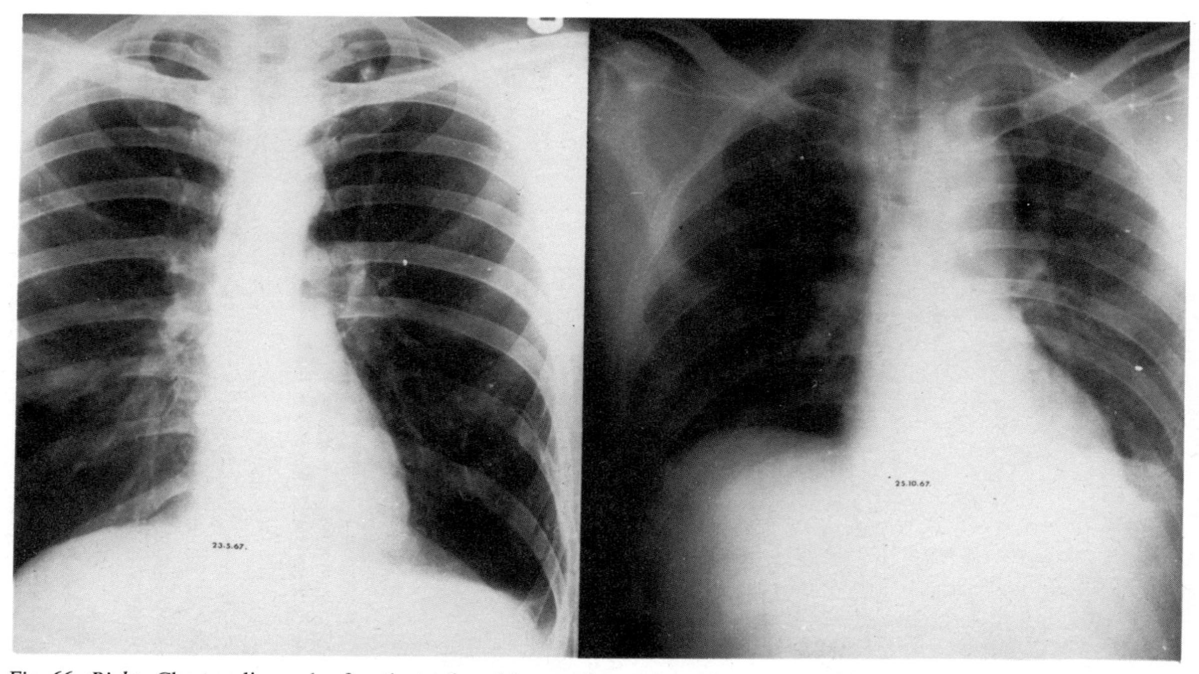

Fig. 66. *Right:* Chest radiograph of patient taken 4 hours after serious motor car accident. When compared with routine chest X-ray taken 5 months prior to the accident (*left*) it is clear that the mediastinal shadow is considerably enlarged.

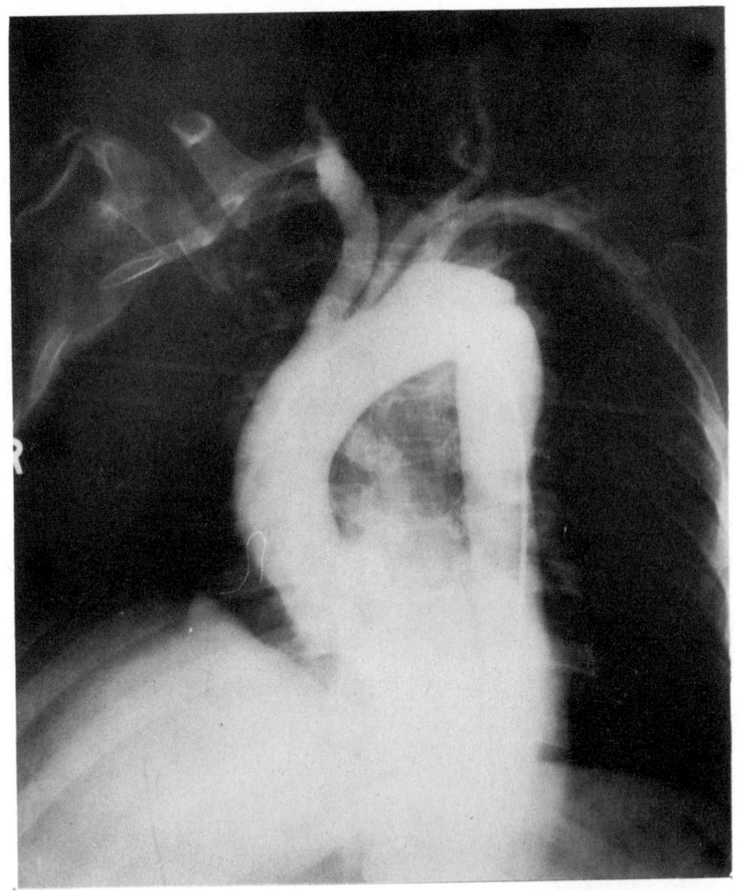

Fig. 67. Aortogram of patient shown in *Fig*. 66 which demonstrates circumferential tear of the aorta at the level of the ligamentum.

period of safe aortic occlusion under these conditions is so unreliable and variable and the risk of ventricular fibrillation during the surface cooling of badly injured people is so high that the use of this technique is no longer advised.

FEMORAL VENOUS-TO-ARTERIAL OXYGENATION

This was described in 1968 in the treatment of 19 patients who underwent resection of aneurysms of the descending aorta or the repair of ruptured aortas (Neville et al., 1968). A large-bore catheter

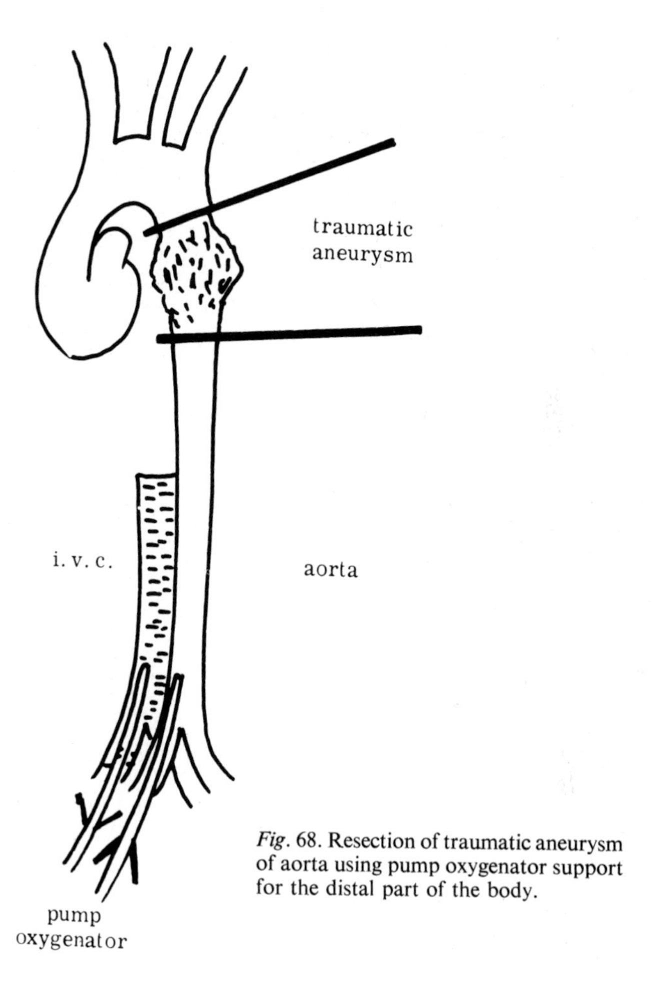

Fig. 68. Resection of traumatic aneurysm of aorta using pump oxygenator support for the distal part of the body.

is inserted into the inferior vena cava via the femoral vein, whence blood is drained into a disposable bubble oxygenator and returned to the femoral artery (*Fig*. 68). This allows a measured perfusion of the lower part of the body during aortic cross-clamping and decompresses the proximal circulation. It has the additional advantage of removing cannulae and tubing from the operative field and avoids cannulation of the left atrium. Although this method does not seem to be in widespread use, it offers an attractive alternative to left atriofemoral by-pass.

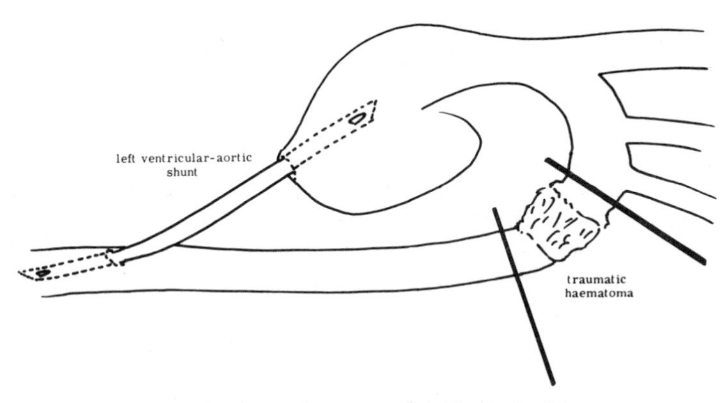

Fig. 69. Diagram of left ventriculo-aortic shunt.

ARTERIAL SHUNTS (*Fig*. 69)

In 1970 Molloy reported the successful repair of ruptured thoracic aorta in 3 patients with the use of a left ventriculo-aortic shunt. A plastic cannula was used, one end of which was inserted into the left ventricle at its apex and the other into the descending thoracic aorta below the site of trauma. The only complication reported was clotting of blood in the cannula on one occasion. The advantages of this method are the avoidance of both heparinization and elaborate by-pass procedures. It is extremely simple and it may well be that it will ultimately be favoured as the procedure of choice in the repair of traumatic rupture of the descending aorta. However, it is probably safer to retain more reliable means of by-pass during the resection of aneurysms.

Kahn (1970) described the use of a temporary plastic shunt inserted at one end into the ascending aorta and at the other into the descending aorta in operations to repair traumatic rupture of the aorta, but reported the occurrence of paraplegia in one patient which may have been due to too small a diameter of shunt. A further report described the use of a shunt from the left subclavian artery to the left femoral artery using a heparin-bonded plastic tube (Gott, 1971).

SURGERY OF ASCENDING AORTA, AORTIC ARCH AND ITS BRANCHES

This is a complicated problem, for in order to resect aneurysms or repair damage of the ascending aorta, the innominate or carotid arteries, some means of protecting the brain from anoxic damage may be required. In rupture of the ascending aorta, full cardiopulmonary bypass may be required, and in damage to the innominate artery localized bypass using Dacron or plastic shunts may be necessary. In order to determine the adequacy of cerebral circulation during these procedures, continuous monitoring with the electro-encephalogram may be helpful. In young patients, however, clamping of one or other of the major head vessels may be undertaken without any form of shunt or cooling, as circulation across the base of the brain may be adequate and this may be established by measuring distal 'stump' pressures during occlusion of these vessels. In complicated injuries, full cardiopulmonary bypass with perfusion, hypothermia and circulatory arrest has been used to facilitate repair.

CASE REPORT (*Figs*. 70, 71)

A 13-year-old girl was admitted following a road traffic accident in which she was a back seat passenger. She sustained concussion and multiple facial lacerations, but on arrival at hospital was conscious, orientated and had no neurological deficit. However, she was noted to have a harsh systolic murmur in the right subclavicular region which radiated into the neck, and the blood pressure in her right arm was lower than her left arm (80/40 compared with 140/70 mmHg). Chest X-ray showed only minimal widening of the mediastinum, but aortography revealed rupture of the innominate artery both at the root and its bifurcation. A median sternotomy was performed and the pericardium was found to contain about 100 ml of altered blood and there was a haematoma at the root of the innominate artery. Gentle palpation revealed complete disruption of the media, the vessel at this point consisting only of a thin layer of adventitia. The innominate artery was then cross-clamped just proximal to its bifurcation into right subclavian and right common carotid arteries, and the distal carotid stump pressure measured. This was found to be 70 mmHg systolic at which time the radial pressure was a mean of 90 mmHg. This indicated that adequate cerebral perfusion was being maintained by the left common carotid and left subclavian and vertebral vessels.

A 12-mm tailored woven Dacron graft was then anastomosed to the ascending aorta using a large Satinsky side-occluding clamp. A further side clamp was then applied to the arch of the aorta at the origin of the innominate artery, taking care not to occlude the left common carotid artery. The origin of the innominate artery was then resected and the defect in the aorta closed with 3/0 Prolene buttressed with Teflon felt. The innominate artery was then resected up to its bifurcation and the distal end of the graft sutured in place. The patient made an excellent recovery, with no neurological or vascular deficit.

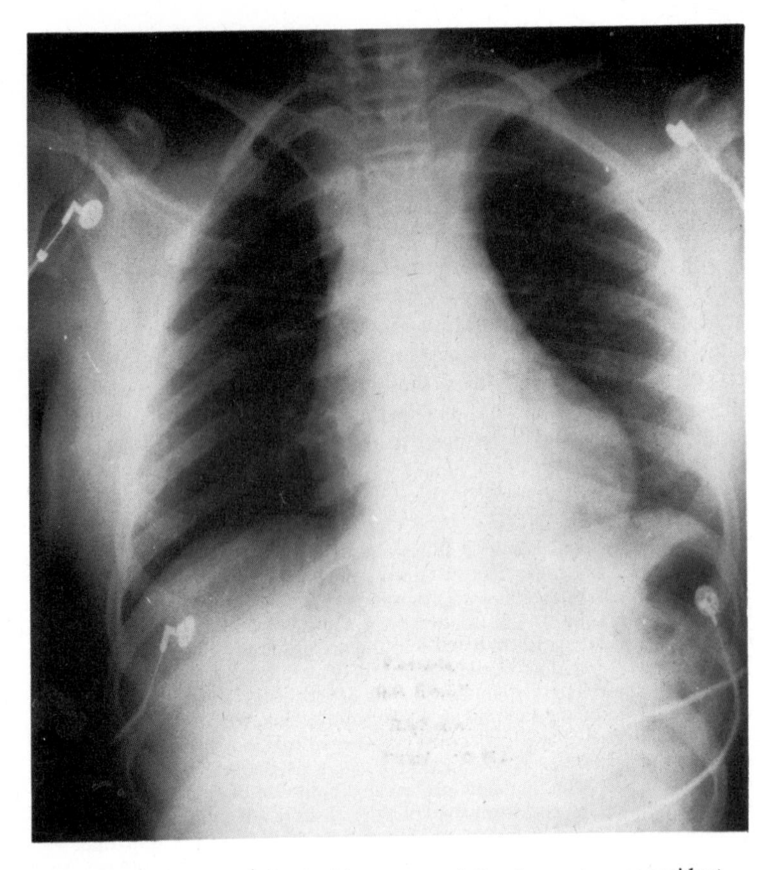

Fig. 70. Traumatic mediastinal haematoma following motor car accident.

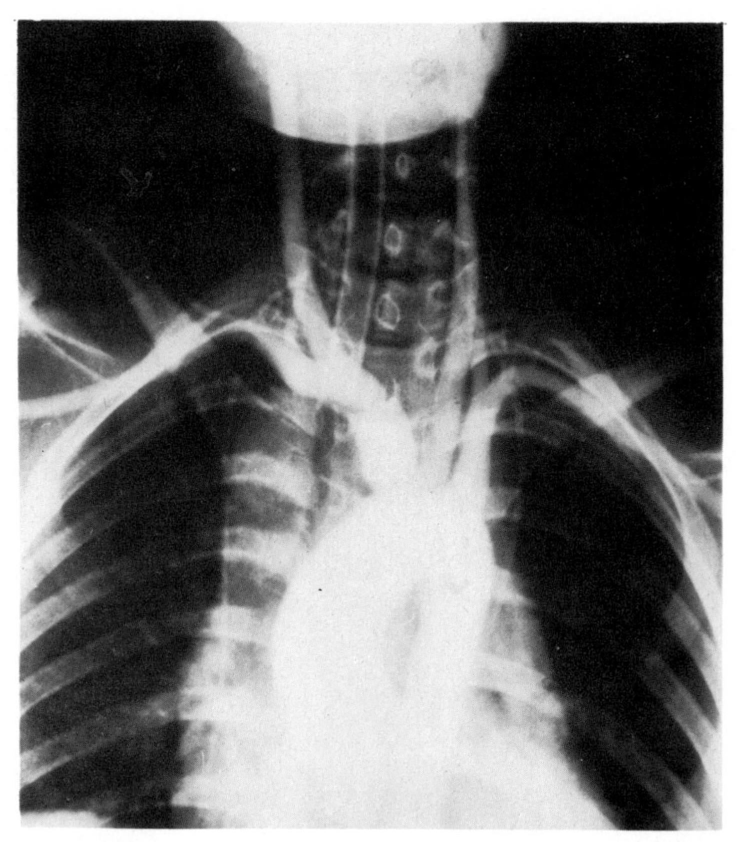

Fig. 71. Aortogram of patient shown in *Fig.* 70 demonstrating rupture of the distal innominate artery.

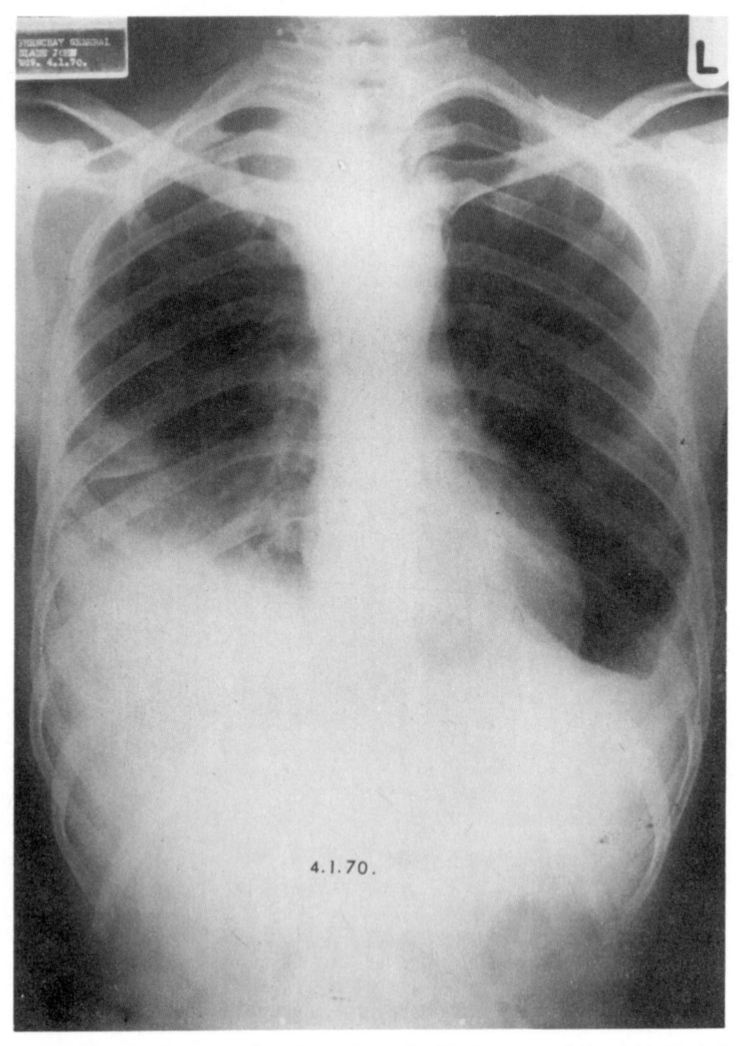

Fig. 72. Chest radiograph of patient admitted with fractures of the right ribs 1–8.

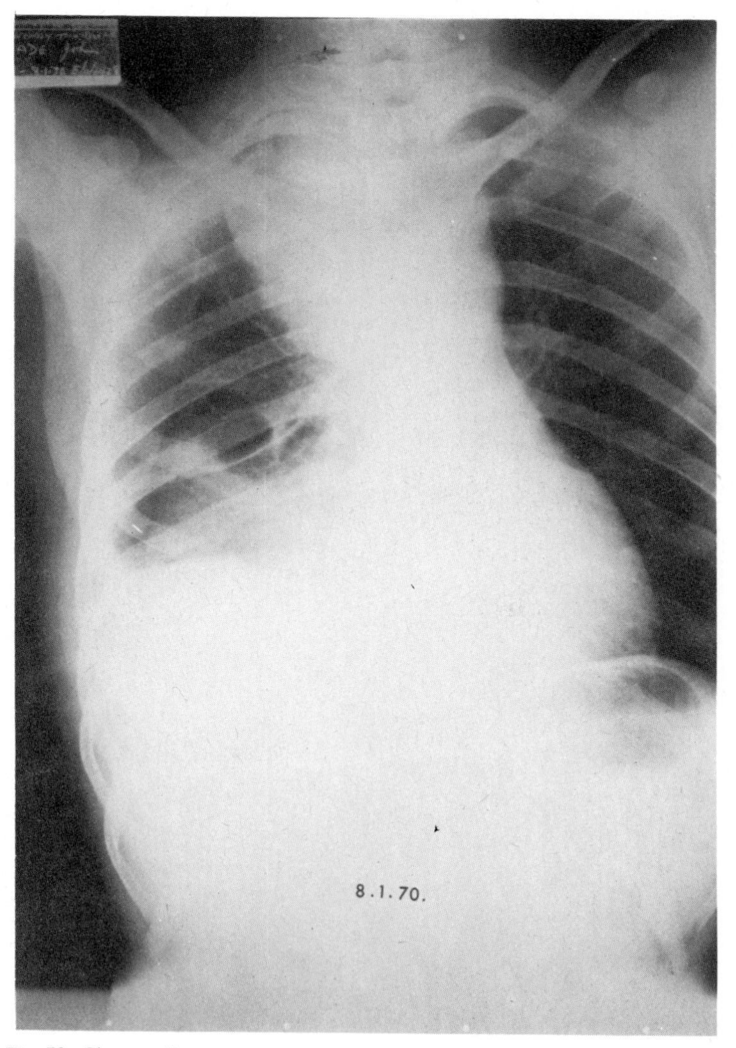

Fig. 73. Chest radiograph of patient shown in *Fig*. 72 4 days following injury. There is now present a large right-sided superior mediastinal mass.

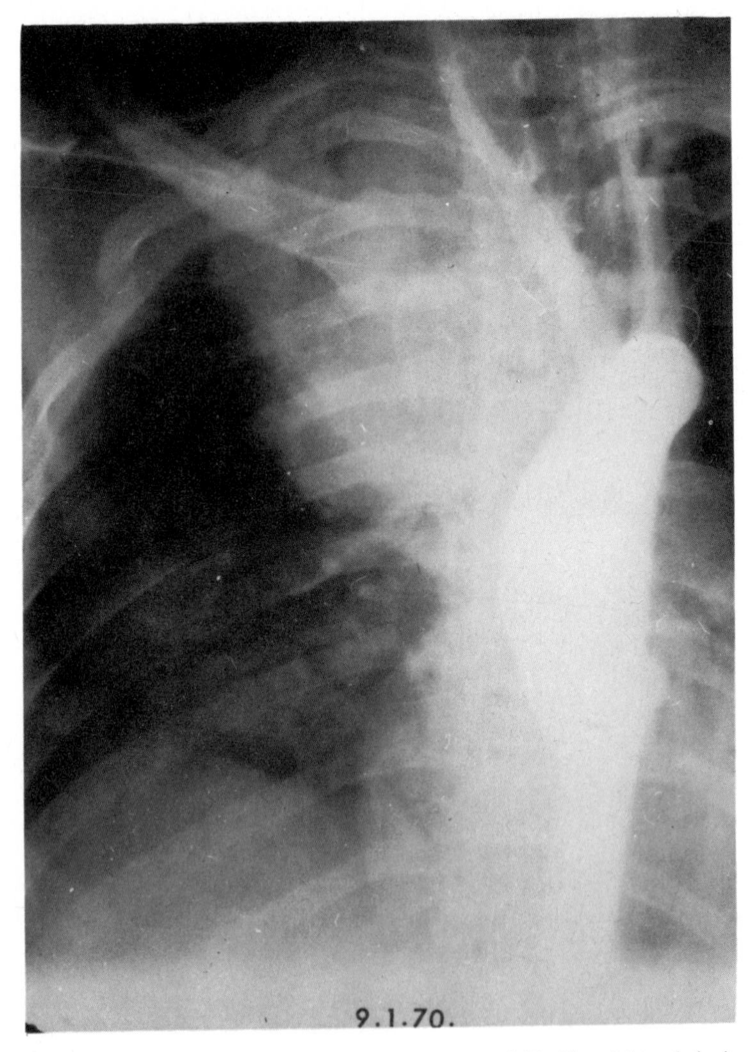

Fig. 74. Aortogram of patient shown in *Figs*. 72 and 73. The right subclavian artery does not fill and it was later confirmed that this artery had been avulsed at its origin from the innominate artery.

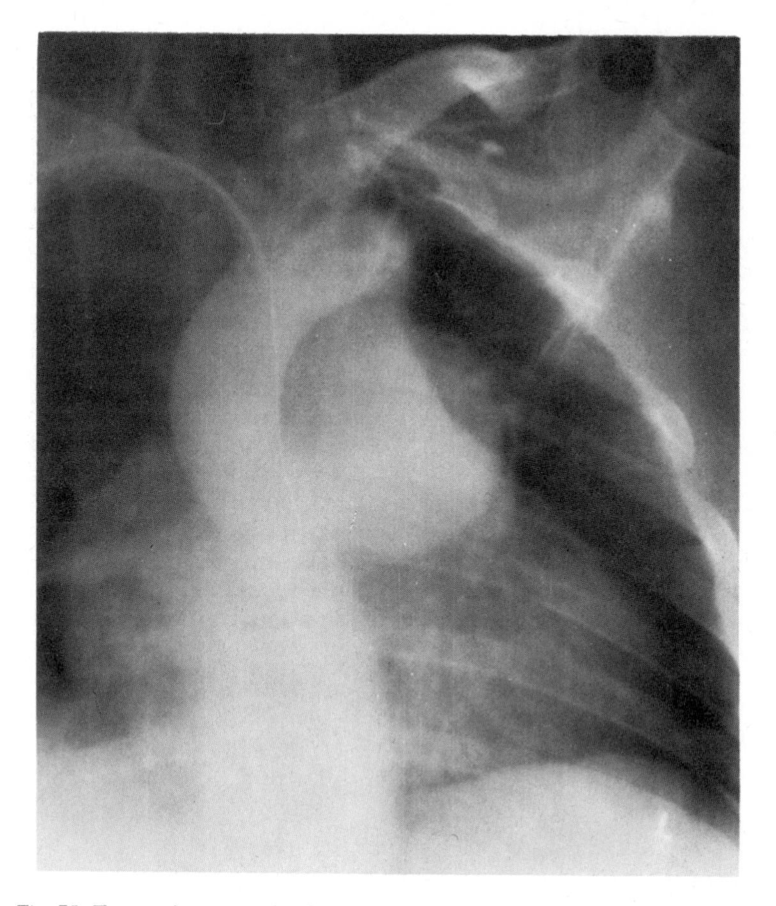

Fig. 75. Traumatic aneurysm of the aorta. This was noted 5 years following a motor vehicle accident and was successfully resected with Dacron graft replacement using left atriofemoral by-pass.

Others have used moderate hypothermia when repairing a ruptured innominate artery and one patient has been reported in whom rupture of the innominate artery was successfully repaired using a combination of cardiopulmonary by-pass and circulatory arrest at 15 °C (Bosher and Freed, 1967).

Others have reported the successful use of profound hypothermia and circulatory arrest in aortic arch repair (Drew et al., 1959; Dumanian et al., 1970). The surgical approach to traumatic rupture of traumatic aneurysms of the right subclavian artery within the chest may be extremely difficult, but a combination of median sternotomy with appropriate extension of the exploration into the right chest and neck provides adequate control (*Figs*. 72, 73 and 74).

CONCLUSIONS

Traumatic rupture of the aorta is by no means rare and an appreciable number of patients are admitted to hospital with this injury. Many still die due primarily to a lack of awareness of the condition or to failure to recognize the tell-tale radiological evidence, for with timely diagnosis the majority of such patients should be saved. Although the progression of events may be so rapid that surgical repair needs to be undertaken by general surgeons at the admitting hospital, these patients, who travel well, are best transferred to centres with appropriate experience and apparatus. Late traumatic aneurysms are by no means benign and their resection should be advised.

Chapter 18

Indications for thoracotomy following chest injuries

Although less than 2 per cent of patients with chest injuries require exploratory thoracotomy, the indications for so doing are well defined and if necessary exploration should not be long delayed. When possible the diagnosis must be supported by appropriate investigations, for unnecessary exploratory thoracotomy in an already badly injured patient may well prejudice survival. With experience, fewer explorations are undertaken, a good example being that of premature and unnecessary thoracotomy for intrathoracic bleeding. The following list of indications will cover many circumstances. In some instances the need for thoracotomy is urgent but in others a period of delay is in order to enable accurate diagnosis to be established.

1. Severe and continued bleeding via chest drainage tubes.
2. Massive haemoptysis associated with parenchymal lung damage.
3. Cardiac tamponade.
4. Uncontrollable pleural air leak.
5. Traumatic rupture of the oesophagus.
6. Open pneumothorax and traumatic thoracotomy.
7. Gross pleural contamination with foreign bodies.
8. Traumatic rupture of the diaphragm.
9. Traumatic rupture of the aorta.
10. Valvular and septal cardiac injuries.

Severe and Continued Bleeding

This has precipitated numerous unnecessary thoracotomies, which is understandable, for the drainage of several units of blood following insertion of an intercostal tube may be quite frightening and the continued drainage of blood may appear to indicate massive bleeding from a major vessel. However, most bleeding from chest wall, diaphragm or pulmonary vessels will cease spontaneously and the mere presence of haemothorax regardless of the amount of blood present does not constitute an absolute indication for thoracotomy. Aspiration and tube drainage will in most instances be followed by re-expansion of the lung and the cessation of bleeding and the emergency will pass following replacement by transfusion. It is difficult to lay down rules in this situation, although if despite adequate drainage a blood loss of more than 500 ml per hour persists for more than 3 hours the need for thoracotomy should be considered. It is important to replace blood loss prior to operation, for general anaesthesia in the presence of serious hypovolaemia may be followed by dangerous hypotension due to the loss of compensatory vasoconstriction associated with anaesthesia. At thoracotomy the sources of bleeding may be the lungs, thoracic wall vessels, diaphragmatic vessels or the great vessels of the mediastinum.

Massive Haemoptysis

This not only endangers the patient from blood loss but is associated with aspiration of blood into the good lung with consequent serious anoxia which, if unrelieved, will be rapidly fatal. From time to time emergency lobectomy is necessary in this situation. If the site of bleeding can be located at bronchoscopy, tamponade of the bronchus with a Fogarty balloon catheter may be effective in isolating the bleeding thus preventing the patient drowning in his own blood.

Pericardial Tamponade

This condition is discussed at length on p. 115, but it must be recognized that with the onset of frank tamponade very little time should be lost before thoracotomy is undertaken. If necessary this should be done within the patient's bed.

Massive Pleural Air Leak with Ruptured Bronchus or Trachea

In the great majority of cases intercostal drainage of pneumothorax is followed by re-expansion of the lung and in those patients in whom air leak persists the loss is not serious. However, from time to time, despite drainage and high volume suction, the lung remains collapsed and serious anoxia develops. In these instances it seems clear that much of the air entering the patient's airway from above is sucked out at once via the drainage tube and that little ventilation is possible. In these circumstances urgent thoracotomy may be required.

Traumatic Rupture of the Oesophagus

This rare injury is an indication for thoracotomy and following confirmation of the diagnosis by contrast radiography exploration should not be long delayed.

Open Pneumothorax and Traumatic Thoracotomy

The presence of these injuries constitutes absolute indications for exploration followed by repair of underlying damage and reconstitution of the chest wall.

Gross Pleural Contamination with Foreign Bodies

These wounds require early débridement and repair of associated damage.

Traumatic Rupture of the Diaphragm

The presence of this injury constitutes an indication for early thoracotomy. From time to time mediastinal displacement and a tension situation is so urgent that immediate thoracotomy within the patient's bed is indicated, but far more frequently more leisurely operation is possible.

Traumatic Rupture of the Aorta

Those patients in whom aortic damage is so severe that immediate thoracotomy is required to arrest haemorrhage are unlikely to survive. Those with radiological mediastinal widening, which is found at aortography to be due to aortic damage, require exploration with appropriate by-pass conditions as soon as the apparatus and surgical team can be assembled.

Valvular and Septal Cardiac Injuries

Those patients in whom valvular or septal injuries are diagnosed have in many instances stabilized sufficiently to allow accurate diagnosis and planned repair, following if necessary a period of treatment of congestive cardiac failure.

Bibliography

Alford B. R., Johnson R. L. and Harris H. H. (1963) Penetrating and perforating injuries of the oesophagus. *Ann. Otol.* **72,** 995.

Ashbaugh D. G. and Petty T. L. (1973) Positive end expiratory pressure. Physiology, indications and contra indications. *J. Thorac. Cardiovasc. Surg.* **65,** 165.

Avery E. E., Morch E. T. and Benson D. W. (1956) Critically crushed chests. A new method of treatment with continuous mechanical hyperventilation to product alkalotic apnea and internal pneumatic stabilization. *J. Thorac. Surg.* **32,** 291.

Barrett N. R. (1946) Spontaneous perforation of the oesophagus. *Thorax* **1,** 48.

Barrett N. R. (1960) Early treatment of 'stove-in' chest. *Lancet* **1,** 293.

Baskett P. J. F. and Bennett J. A. (1971) Pain relief in hospital: the more widespread use of nitrous oxide. *Br. Med. J.* **2,** 509–511.

Beall A. C. jun. (1960) Penetrating wounds of the aorta. *Am. J. Surg.* **99,** 770.

Beall A. C. jun., Hamit H. F., Cooley D. A. and DeBakey M. E. (1965) Surgical management of traumatic intracardiac lesions. *J. Trauma* **5,** 133.

Beall A. C. jun., Ochsner J. L., Morris G. C., Cooley D. A. and DeBakey M. E. (1961) Penetrating wounds of the heart. *J. Trauma* **1,** 195.

Belsey R. H. R. (1965) Reconstruction of the oesophagus with left colon. *J. Thorac. Cardiovasc. Surg.* **49,** 33.

Bickford J. (1974) Chest injuries: review of five years' experience. *Thorax* **29,** 269.

Biermer A. (1863) *Schweiz. z. Heilk.* **2,** 146.

Billy L. J., Amato J. J. and Rich M. M. (1971) Aortic injuries in Vietnam. *Surgery* **70,** 385.

Bishop C. O., Miller A. C. and Burch B. H. (1960) Fracture of the bronchial tree following blunt chest trauma. *West. J. Surg. Obstet. Gynec.* **68,** 345.

Bland E. F. and Beebe G. W. (1966) Missiles in the heart: a twenty year follow-up report of World War II cases. *N. Engl. J. Med.* **274,** 1039.

Bloodwell R. D., Hallman G. L. and Cooley D. A. (1966) Aneurysm of the ascending aorta with valvular insufficiency: surgical management. *Arch. Surg.* **92,** 588.

Boerhaave H. (1724) Quoted by Barrett N. R. (1946).

Borrie J. (1969) Congenital complete absence of left pericardium. *Thorax* **24,** 756.

Borrie J. and Lichter I. (1974) Pericardial rupture from blunt chest trauma. *Thorax* **29,** 329.

Bosher L. H. and Freed T. A. (1967) The surgical treatment of traumatic avulsion of the innominate artery. *J. Thorac. Cardiovasc. Surg.* **54,** 732.

Boxall R. (1886) Incomplete pericardial sac: escape of heart into left pleural cavity. *Trans. Obst. Soc. Lond.* **28,** 209.

Carlsson E. and Silander T. (1963) Rupture of the subclavian and innominate artery due to non-penetrating trauma of the chest. *Acta Chir. Scand.* **125,** 294.

Clarke D. B. (1975) Personal communication.

CLEVELAND R. J., BENFIELD J. R., NEMHAUSER G. M. and LOWER R. R. (1968) Management of penetrating wounds of the heart. *Arch. Surg.* **97,** 517.

CONNOLLY J. E., WAKABAYASHI A., GERMAN J. C., STEMMER E. A. and SERRES E. J. (1971) Clinical experience with pulsatile left heart bypass without anticoagulation for thoracic aneurysm. *J. Thorac. Cardiovasc. Surg.* **62,** 568.

COOLEY D. A. (1969) Personal communication.

COOLEY D. A., DEBAKEY M. E. and MORRIS G. C. (1957) Controlled extracorporeal circulation in surgical treatment of aortic aneurysm. *Ann. Surg.* **146,** 473.

CRAWFORD E. S., FENSTERMACHER J. M., RICHARDSON W. and SANDIFORD F. (1970) Reappraisal of adjuncts to avoid ischaemia in the treatment of thoracic aortic aneurysms. *Surgery* **67,** 182.

CRAWFORD E. S. and RUBIO P. A. (1973) Reappraisal of adjuncts to avoid ischaemia in the treatment of aneurysms of descending thoracic aorta. *J. Thorac. Cardiovasc. Surg.* **66,** 693.

DEBAKEY M. E. (1968) Personal communication.

DEMEULES J. E., CRAMER G. and PERRY J. F. (1971) Rupture of aorta and great vessels due to blunt thoracic trauma. *J. Thorac. Cardiovasc. Surg.* **61,** 438.

DEMUTH W. E. jun. and ZINSSER H. F. jun. (1965) Myocardial contusion. *Arch. Int. Med.* **115,** 434.

DREW C. E. and ANDERSON I. M. (1959) Profound hypothermia in cardiac surgery: report of 3 cases. *Lancet* **1,** 748.

DREW C. E., KEEN G. and BENAZON D. B. (1959) Profound hypothermia. *Lancet* **1,** 745.

DUMANIAN A. V., HOEKSEMA T. D., SANTSCHI D. R., GREENWALD J. H. and FRAHM C. J. (1970) Profound hypothermia and circulatory arrest in the treatment of traumatic aortic aneurysms. *J. Thorac. Cardiovasc. Surg.* **59,** 541.

EARLE P. (1841) Case of Thomas Tipple. *Am. J. Med. Sci.* **2,** 113.

EISEMAN B. and RAINER W. G. (1958) Clinical management of post traumatic rupture of the thoracic aorta. *J. Thorac. Surg.* **35,** 347.

ELKIN D. C. and CAMPBELL R. E. (1951) Cardiac tamponade, treatment by aspiration. *Ann. Surg.* **133,** 623.

GERBODE F., BRAIMBRIDGE M., OSBORN J. J., HOOD M. and FRENCH S. (1957) Traumatic thoracic aneurysms: treatment by resection and grafting with the use of an extracorporeal bypass. *Surgery* **42,** 975.

GIBSON L. D., CARTER R. and HINSHAW D. B. (1962) Surgical significance of sternal fractures. *Surg. Gynecol. Obstet.* **114,** 443.

GOORWICH J. (1955) Traumatic chylothorax and thoracic duct ligation. Case report and review of literature. *J. Thorac. Surg.* **29,** 467.

GOTT V. L. (1971) Discussion following paper by CONNOLLY et al. (1971).

GRIFFITH J. L. (1949) Traumatic fracture of the left main bronchus. *Thorax* **4,** 105.

GRILLO H. C., COOPER J. D., GEFFIN B. and PONTOPPIDAN H. (1971) A low pressure cuff for tracheostomy tubes to minimize tracheal injury. *J. Thorac. Cardiovasc. Surg.* **62,** 898.

GUEST J. L. jun., HALL D. P., YEH T. J. and ELLISON R. G. (1965) Late manifestations of trauma to the pericardium. *Surg. Gynecol. Obstet.* **120,** 787.

GUILFOIL P. H. and DOYLE J. T. (1953) Traumatic cardiac septal defect: report of a case in which the diagnosis is established by cardiac catheterization. *J. Thorac. Surg.* **25,** 510.

HARDY J. D. and WILLIAMS R. D. (1967) Penetrating heart wounds: analysis of 12 consecutive cases individualized without mortality. *Ann. Surg.* **166,** 228.

HARKEN D. E. (1946) Foreign bodies in, and in relation to, the thoracic blood vessels and heart. *Surg. Gynecol. Obstet.* **83,** 117.

HARLEY H. R. S. (1971) Laryngo-tracheal obstruction complicating tracheostomy or endotracheal intubation with assisted respiration. *Thorax* **26,** 493.

HILL D. J., DE LEVAL M. R., FALLAT R. J., BRAMSON M. L., EBENHART R. C., SCHULTE H. D., OSBORN J. J., BARBER R. and GERBODE F. (1972) Acute respiratory insufficiency. Treatment with prolonged extracorporeal circulation. *J. Thorac. Cardiovasc. Surg.* **64,** 551.

HILL D. J., O'BRIEN T. G., MURRAY J. J., DONTIGNY L., BRAMSON M. L., OSBORN J. J. and GERBODE F. (1972) Prolonged extracorporeal oxygenation for acute post traumatic respiratory failure (shock lung syndrome). *N. Engl. J. Med.* **286,** 629.

HILL L. L. (1900) Wounds of the heart with a report of 17 cases of heart suture. *Med. Rec.* **58,** 921.

HUGHES J. T. (1964) Spinal cord infarction due to aortic trauma. *Br. Med. J.* **2,** 356.

KAHN D. R. (1970) Discussion following paper by CRAWFORD et al., 1970.

KEEN G. (1968) The surgical management of old oesophageal perforations. *J. Thorac. Cardiovasc. Surg.* **56,** 531.

KEEN G. (1972) Closed injuries of the thoracic aorta. *Ann. R. Coll. Surg.* **51,** 137.

KINSELLA T. J. and JOHNSRUD L. W. (1947) Traumatic rupture of the bronchus. *J. Thorac. Surg.* **16,** 571.

KRINITZKI S. I. (1928) *Virchows Arch.* (*Pathol. Anat.*) **266,** 815.

LAMPSON R. S. (1948) Traumatic chylothorax: a review of the literature and report of a case treated by mediastinal ligation of the thoracic duct. *J. Thorac. Surg.* **17,** 778.

LIGHTWOOD R. G. and CLELAND W. P. (1974) Cervical lung hernia. *Thorax* **29,** 349.

LLOYD J. R., HEYDINGER D. K., KLASSEN K. P. and ROETTIG L. C. (1958) Rupture of the main bronchi in closed chest injury. A reproduction in the experimental animal. *Arch. Surg.* **77,** 597.

LUCIDO J. L. and WALL C. A. (1963) Rupture of the diaphragm due to blunt trauma. *Arch. Surg.* **86,** 989.

LYONS C. and PERKINS R. (1958) Resection of a left ventricular aneurysm secondary to cardiac stab wound. *Ann. Surg.* **147,** 256.

MAHAFFEY D. E., CREECH O., BOREN H. G. and DEBAKEY M. E. (1956) Traumatic rupture of the left main bronchus successfully repaired eleven years after injury. *J. Thorac. Surg.* **32,** 312.

MALONEY J. V., SCHMUTZER J. K. and EKKEHART R. (1961) Paradoxical respiration and *Pendelluft*. *J. Thorac. Cardiovasc. Surg.* **41,** 291.

MALONEY J. V. and SPENCER F. C. (1956) The non-operative treatment of traumatic chylothorax. *Surgery* **40,** 121.

MARABLE S. A. and MALONEY J. V. (1963) Bilateral transfixion injury of the thorax. *J. Thorac. Cardiovasc. Surg.* **45,** 161.

MATTOX K. L., BEALL A. C. jun., JORDAN G. L. jun. and DEBAKEY M. E. (1974) Cardiorraphy in the emergency center. *J. Thorac. Cardiovasc. Surg.* **68,** 886.

MICHELSON E. and ROQUE A. H. (1968) Cervical tracheo-oesophageal fistula due to steering wheel injury. *Ann. Thorac. Surg.* **5,** 178.

MOLLOY P. J. (1970) Repair of the ruptured thoracic aorta using left ventriculo-aortic support. *Thorax* **25,** 213.

MOORE B. P. (1975) Operative stabilisation of non penetrating chest injuries. *J. Thorac. Cardiovasc. Surg.* **70,** 619.

MURRAY G. F., BRAWLEY R. K. and GOTT V. L. (1971) Reconstruction of the innominate artery by means of a temporary heparin-coated shunt bypass. *J. Thorac. Cardiovasc. Surg.* **62,** 34.

NACLEREO E. A. (1964) Penetrating wounds of the heart: experience with 249 patients. *Dis. Chest* **46,** 1.

NEVILLE W. E., COX W. D., LEININGER B. and PIFARRE R. (1968) Resection of the thoracic aorta with femoral vein to femoral artery perfusion with oxygenation. *J. Thorac. Cardiovasc. Surg.* **56,** 39.

NICHOLLS F. (1728) *Philos. Trans. R. Soc. Lond.* **35,** 440.

OPPENHEIM F. (1918) *Münch. Med. Wochenschr.* **65,** 1234.

OVERSTREET J. W. and OCHSNER A. (1955) Traumatic rupture of the oesophagus. Report of 13 cases. *J. Thorac. Surg.* **30,** 164.

PARMLEY L. F., MANION W. C., MATTINGLY T. W. and JAHNKE E. J. (1958) Nonpenetrating traumatic injury of the aorta. *Circulation* **17,** 1086.

PARMLEY L. F., MATTINGLY T. W. and MANION W. C. (1958) Penetrating wounds of the heart and aorta. *Circulation* **17,** 953.

PASSARO E. and PACE W. G. (1959) Traumatic rupture of the aorta. *Surgery* **46,** 787.

PIERCE E. C., DABBS G. H. and RAWSON F. L. (1958) Isolated rupture of the ventricular septum due to nonpenetrating trauma. *Arch. Surg.* **77,** 87.

RAVITCH M. M. and BLALOCK A. (1949) Aspiration of blood from pericardium in treatment of acute cardiac tamponade after injury: further experience, with report of cases. *Arch. Surg.* **58,** 463.

REHN L. (1897) Ueber Penetrierende Herzwunden und Herznaht. *Arch. Klin. Chir.* **55,** 315.

REHN L. (1907) Zur Chirurgie des Herzens und des Herzbeutels. *Arch. Klin. Chir.* **83,** 723.

REUL G. R. jun., RUBIO P. A. and BEALL A. C. (1974) Surgical management of acute injuries of the thoracic aorta. *J. Thorac. Cardiovasc. Surg.* **67,** 272.

RICE W. G. and WITTSTRUCK K. P. (1951) Acute hypertension and delayed traumatic rupture of the aorta. *J.A.M.A.* **147,** 915.

ROBB D. (1963) Traumatic diaphragmatic hernia into the pericardium. *Br. J. Surg.* **50,** 664.

ROBIN E., BELAMARIE J., THOMAS N. W., ARBULU A. and SUNILENDU G. N. (1974) Consequences of total tricuspid valvulectomy without prosthetic replacement in treatment of *Pseudomonas* endocarditis. *J. Thorac. Cardiovasc. Surg.* **68,** 461.

SAILER S. (1942) Dissecting aneurysm of the aorta. *Arch. Pathol.* **33,** 704.

SAMPSON P. C. (1955) In Discussion of RICHARDS V. and COHN R. B.: Rupture of the thoracic trachea and major bronchi following closed injury to the chest. *Am. J. Surg.* **90,** 253.

SANDOR F. (1967) Incidence and significance of traumatic mediastinal haematoma. *Thorax* **22,** 43.

SANGER P. W. (1945) Evacuation hospital experiences with war wounds and injuries of the chest. *Ann. Surg.* **122,** 147.

SCANNELL J. G. (1951) Rupture of bronchus following closed injury to the chest: report of a case treated by immediate thoracotomy and repair. *Ann. Surg.* **133,** 127.

SEVITT S. (1968) Fatal road accidents, injuries, complications and causes of death in 250 subjects. *Br. J. Surg.* **55,** 481.

SLANEY G., ASHTON F. and ABRAMS L. D. (1966) Traumatic rupture of the aorta. *Br. J. Surg.* **53,** 361.

Sondergaard T. (1970) Personal communication.
Spencer F. C., Guerin P. F., Blake H. A. and Bahnson H. T. (1961) A report of 15 patients with traumatic rupture of the thoracic aorta. *J. Thorac. Cardiovasc. Surg.* **41,** 1.
Steichen F. M., Dargan E. L., Efron G., Pearlman D. M. and Weil P. H. (1971) A graded approach to the management of penetrating wounds to the heart. *Arch. Surg.* **103,** 574.
Steinberg I. (1957) Chronic traumatic aneurysm of the thoracic aorta. *N. Engl. J. Med.* **257,** 913.
Strassman G. (1947) Traumatic rupture of the aorta. *Am. Heart. J.* **33,** 508.
Stryker W. A. (1948) Traumatic saccular aneurysm of the thoracic aorta. *Am. J. Clin. Pathol.* **18,** 152.
Swan H., Forsee J. H. and Goyette E. M. (1952) Foreign bodies in the heart. *Ann. Surg.* **135,** 314.
Taber R. E. (1970) Discussion of paper by Crawford E. S. et al. (1970).
Teare D. (1951) Post-mortem examinations on air crash victims. *Br. Med. J.* **2,** 707.
Webb A. (1848) *Pathologia Indica or the Anatomy of Indian Diseases*, 2nd ed. Calcutta. (Biermer C. T. N. A. (1863) *Schweiz. z. Heilk.* **2,** 150.)
Williams K. R. and Burford T. H. (1963) The management of chylothorax in relation to trauma. *J. Trauma* **3,** 317.
Windsor H. M. and Dwyer B. (1961) The crushed chest. *Thorax* **16,** 3.
Worman L. W., Hurley J. D., Pemberton A. H. and Narodick B. G. (1962) Rupture of the oesophagus from external blunt trauma. *Arch. Surg.* **85,** 333.
Wren H. B., Texada P. J. and Krementz E. T. (1962) Traumatic rupture of the diaphragm. *J. Trauma* **2,** 117.

Index